£12.95

CLINICAL FINALS AND HOW TO PASS THEM

For Churchill Livingstone:

Publisher: Laurence Hunter
Project Editor: Janice Urquhart
   Copy Editor: Jennifer Bew
Project Controller: Nancy Arnott
Design Direction: Erik Bigland
Page Layout: Kate Walshaw

CLINICAL FINALS
AND HOW TO PASS THEM

KEVIN P. HANRETTY MD MRCOG
Consultant Obstetrician and Gynaecologist,
The Queen Mother's Hospital, Glasgow, UK

TOM TURNER FRCP
Consultant Paediatrician,
The Royal Hospital for Sick Children, Glasgow, UK

JOHN R. McGREGOR MD FRCS
Consultant Surgeon,
Crosshouse Hospital, Kilmarnock, UK

STUART HOOD MRCP
Registrar in Cardiology,
The Royal Infirmary, Glasgow, UK

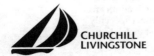

CHURCHILL
LIVINGSTONE

EDINBURGH LONDON MADRID MELBOURNE NEW YORK SAN FRANCISCO
AND TOKYO 1998

CHURCHILL LIVINGSTONE
Medical Division of Pearson Professional Limited

Distributed in the United States of America by
Churchill Livingstone Inc., 650 Avenue of the Americas,
New York, N.Y. 10011, and by associated companies,
branches and representatives throughout the world.

© Pearson Professional Limited 1998

First published 1998

ISBN 0 443 05923 3

British Library of Cataloguing in Publication Data
A catalogue record for this book is available from the
British Library.

Library of Congress Cataloging in Publication Data
A catalogue record for this book is available from the
Library of Congress

Medical knowledge is constantly changing. As new
information becomes available, changes in treatment,
procedures, equipment and the use of drugs become
necessary. The authors and the publishers have, as far as it
is possible, taken care to ensure that the information given
in this text is accurate and up to date. However, readers are
strongly advised to confirm that the information, especially
with regard to drug usage, complies with latest legislation
and standards of practice.

The
publisher's
policy is to use
**paper manufactured
from sustainable forests**

Produced by Longman Asia Ltd, Hong Kong
EPC/01

PREFACE

The move towards day-care management in all disciplines in medicine has led to a decrease in the numbers of patients available for bedside teaching. This has resulted in a reduction in the opportunities for preparation and development of the specific techniques required to pass clinical examinations. Further, most medical school curricula remain system-based. However both clinical practice and clinical examination technique are problem-based, and the authors, who are experienced in both organizing and examining in the Final MB examinations, saw a need for a handbook which would aid students in their preparation for the clinical examinations.

The changing role of the junior hospital doctor has also led to a reduction in the opportunities for registrars hoping to cultivate their own teaching skills and they may find this handbook useful when beginning to develop this expertise. Finally, it is hoped that this handbook may help students to develop their talents in order to achieve the principal aim of being good doctors.

Glasgow 1998   K. P. H.

CONTENTS

1. INTRODUCTION
1

2. MEDICINE
11

HISTORY AND EXAMINATION IN MEDICINE 11
THE CASES 13
  Cerebrovascular disorders 13
  Chest pain 16
  Diabetes mellitus 20
  Finger on the pulse 22
  Hypertension 24
  Cardiac murmurs 26
  Dyspnoea 27
  Skin disease 31
  Sore joints 34
  The patient with weight loss/debility 36
  Blackouts 38
  Dementia 41
  Diarrhoea/change in bowel habit 42
  Jaundice (medical aspects) 45
  Neurological patients (excluding 'blackouts') 48
  Thyroid patients (medical aspects) 50
  Anaemic patients 52
  Headache 55
  Renal failure (medical aspects) 57

AN A–Z IN MEDICINE
Questions   60
Answers   67

3. SURGERY   79

HISTORY AND EXAMINATION IN SURGERY   79
THE CASES   86
Altered bowel habit (surgical aspects)   86
Herniae   88
Jaundice (surgical aspects)   93
Rectal bleeding   96
Skin lesions   97
Stomas   102
Upper abdominal pain   106
Varicose veins   110
Leg ulcers   113
Neck lumps (excluding the thyroid)   115
Scrotal lumps   119
Thyroid patients   121
Toenails   124
Breast lumps   126
Dysphagia   130
Equipment   131
Orthopaedic cases   135
Perioperative care   143
Peripheral vascular disease   147
X-rays   153
Aneurysmal arterial disease   156
Renal failure (surgical aspects)   158

AN A–Z IN SURGERY

Questions   161

Answers   169

4. GYNAECOLOGY   181

HISTORY AND EXAMINATION IN GYNAECOLOGY   181

THE CASES   183

Contraception/sterilization   183

Menorrhagia   185

Chronic pelvic pain   188

Hormone replacement treatment (HRT)   190

Infertility   192

Postmenopausal bleeding   194

Prolapse   197

Urinary incontinence   199

Intermenstrual bleeding/abnormal smear   201

Vaginal discharge   204

Vulval mass/pruritus vulvae   206

Pelvic mass   208

Recurrent abortion   211

5. OBSTETRICS   215

HISTORY AND EXAMINATION IN OBSTETRICS   215

THE CASES   220

Multiple pregnancy   220

Normal pregnancy   222

Post-dates pregnancy   224

Pre-eclampsia   225

Previous caesarean section 229
Small-for-dates (SFD) 232
Antepartum haemorrhage (APH) 235
Breech presentation 238
Large-for-dates 242
Medical disorders in pregnancy
 (excluding diabetes) 244
Preterm premature rupture of the membranes 246
Previous postpartum haemorrhage 248
Diabetes in pregnancy 250
Previous fetal loss/abnormality 252
Rhesus disease 254

AN A–Z IN OBSTETRICS AND GYNAECOLOGY

Questions 257
Answers 263

6. PAEDIATRICS

271

HISTORY AND EXAMINATION IN PAEDIATRICS 271
THE CASES 280

Cardiac disease 280
Developmental delay 282
Neurological disorders 284
The scrawny/small child 284
The breathless child 286
Dysmorphism 288
Lumps and bumps 288
Skin problems 289
Painful joint(s) 290

AN A–Z IN PAEDIATRICS

Questions 292
Answers 298

INTRODUCTION

Clinical and oral examinations form a fundamental part of the assessment of your competence at every stage of your clinical undergraduate training. Unfortunately, the performance of candidates in clinical final examinations can be blighted by a poor showing in these areas, and ironically the performance in clinicals and orals often does not reflect either their knowledge or their competence.

You will already have encountered colleagues who do well in written examinations but badly when presented with a real patient. Alternatively you meet people who come out of an examination and complain about how difficult either the cases or the examiners were, when neither is necessarily true. In undergraduate examinations the examiners' aim is to identify that you have met the standards required to practise as a doctor in the supervised post of Junior House Officer. This is a heavy responsibility for the examiners. However, it is important to remember that they really are trying to pass you rather than fail you. You will become bored by the number of times people tell you this, but it is actually true. In other words, defeat in the final MB examination usually results from 'own goals' rather than some enormously difficult case. All students should be able to pass their clinical exams. Acceptance into medical school should mean that you certainly have the intellectual capacity. Why is it, therefore, that some candidates still fail? One answer is simply

1

lack of effort, but we will assume you are not in that category. Basically, success depends on learning the techniques of presentation peculiar to clinical exams. The purpose of this handbook is to help with how you might do this. It is *not* a textbook and not intended as such, but consists of a general introduction to the aspects of history and examination particular to each of the principal disciplines in the finals: medicine, surgery, obstetrics and gynaecology and paediatrics. These are followed by a number of different cases with which you might be presented in the exam. It is well to remember that some poor registrar, with varying degrees of good grace, has been landed with the task of finding cases for the clinical part of the examination, and it is not always possible for him or her to find good cases.

The layout of the cases described here usually begins with a definition, since the commonest starting question for any case is: '… and what exactly do you mean by pre-eclampsia/ inflammatory bowel disease/dyspnoea/failure to thrive?' etc. The number of candidates in these circumstances in clinical and oral examinations who stand opened-mouthed for some moments is disappointing. Rote learning is currently being discouraged, but the inability to give a straightforward definition of a common clinical condition may well constitute an own goal – or at least time wasting – and psychologically it is a bad way to introduce yourself to the examiners.

Each case will be given an indication of the likelihood of that type of case appearing in the exam. This can only be indicative, since certain conditions – for example thalassaemias – may only be seen commonly in larger metropolitan centres. There are five categories: very unlikely, unlikely, possible, likely and very likely. This will apply to the type of case and also to the different possible diagnoses. For example, it may be very likely that you will be presented with a breathless child but only possible that you might see a case of bronchiolitis. Remember, some candidates may still meet cases which would be considered unlikely in the exam. View this as an opportunity to shine rather than terrible luck!

The likelihood will be indicated as follows:	
Very unlikely	★
Unlikely	★★
Possible	★★★
Likely	★★★★
Very likely	★★★★★

The next section for each case will usually relate to the relevant features you might either identify or exclude in the history. It is not the intention here to describe how to take a history: you should have sorted that out by now. It is intended to highlight for you the parts of the history which you should emphasize for the examiners.

Similarly, the next section, on clinical examination, serves to point out the particular findings of relevance in these cases. In most medical schools the examination comprises a bedside examination followed by an oral examination based on the case you have just seen. In addition to the long case, depending on the specialty and the medical school, you may also be presented with short cases which require that you identify specific clinical signs.

In the oral component of the examination you may be asked anything about the discipline and – if you are unlucky – may be asked on topics covered in your preclinical years, such as physiology or anatomy.

Slides and 'pots' may be presented to you for comment.

At the end of each section on examination technique for individual cases is a section on 'facts'. These are intended as little 'tasters' so that you can go back to the textbooks and find out more. Remember, this is not a textbook, but it can nudge you into looking things up. Other facts are included just for general interest. Some of these items lend themselves to particular questions, and you might care to imagine which might reasonably be asked about in your examination.

Discussion points may follow and you might again consider which might reasonably be raised in the examination.

PREPARING FOR THE CLINICAL EXAMINATION

Already you have met people who you know had absolutely every word in the standard textbooks off by heart, and frightened you over coffee by their apparent knowledge. These are sometimes the ones who say 'Oh I've not even begun to study yet', when you know they were up all last night memorizing stuff. Most of these people do obnoxiously well throughout medical school, but a proportion fall at the hurdle of clinical/oral examinations. One of their problems is that the questions asked are often not the type that can be answered by regurgitating a paragraph from a textbook. Usually you rely on being able to synthesize an answer from a variety of sources, the most important of which is your clinical experience. Candidates who have been around the wards learn as much by osmosis from those around them as they do from books.

Medicine is bedevilled by jargon, and an ability to use this is worth acquiring. Remember that the function of jargon is to communicate ideas efficiently, and not to confuse patients or to set you apart by its exclusiveness. Remember also that some examiners object to excessive use of jargon and to some abbreviations: some consultants prefer to avoid terms such as CCF or COAD, but you should certainly be familiar with them and comfortable in their use.

Many of the elements of clinical and viva examinations resemble concert performances. It is useful to consider how a performer prepares himself. The first method is rehearsal, and the value of mock exams cannot be overemphasized.

However, on the day a performer should look the part.

Personal presentation

Do not be insulted if this is too obvious to you. Some candidates still present themselves as slovenly, and although you might not agree with your examiners' ideas of sartorial elegance you will influence their approach to you by your appearance. Conservative dress is the rule, with a dark suit, plain black shoes and a non-club tie. Women do not usually need to be given direction in how to present themselves, but the rule about suits is still a useful one.

Consider how you form impressions of people you never speak to. Even just sitting on the train or on a bus, you make assumptions about those around you. Whether those assumptions are in any way justified is exceedingly doubtful, but think about how readily you form them.

It is likely that the first time the examiners see you at the clinical exam you will be introduced by the invigilator, or the examiners might introduce themselves, or even shake hands. Do not be taken aback by this show of humanity, but remember that they will already have formed an impression of you. Thus, for example, your stance is terribly important. You need not stand to attention, but certain postures imply a lack of respect for the examiners: leaning against a handy radiator with your legs crossed at the ankles is definitely to be avoided, as is folding your arms in the presence of the examiners. In body language terms this is definitely not to be recommended. The impression given by such a posture is that you are putting up barriers or resisting questions. Even if you think you never do this, ask your colleagues. Better still, if you can arrange a mock examination see if someone will videotape it for you. You will be amazed at how often you bring your hands to your ears or mouth, or adopt mannerisms of which you are unaware but which become pronounced under stress and which can annoy examiners.

You should learn which posture you are comfortable in. Some candidates, for example, don't know what to do with their hands when being asked questions, and it is possible to become quite clumsy in such a situation. You will usually have been given a clipboard with paper upon which to make notes. Keep these in your hands. This is helpful for two reasons: the first is that it allows you to refresh your memory occasionally, and the second is that it stops you scratching your nose or eyebrows etc. Do not read from your notes as if you have a short-term memory defect – they are there to act as prompts, not as a script for your case history.

You will be asked to present your case and different examiners will expect different styles of presentation. Particular styles for each specialty are suggested in each section, but to some extent it does not matter how you present your case as long as it is logical. Practise speaking much more slowly than you are accustomed to. Often candidates speak very rapidly indeed, and it can be difficult for examiners to identify that your perceptive, incisive comments are not just babble. This should be commented on by people helping you with mock cases.

The good candidate should be able to anticipate at least some of the more likely questions. For example, if in gynaecology you have presented a case of postmenopausal bleeding, it is sensible to anticipate a question such as 'What are the causes of postmenopausal bleeding?' or 'How should such a case be managed?'

Some points about answering questions in the clinical exam need some emphasis, and this relates to the appropriate use of words. For example, the staging of all malignancies has fixed definitions, but other conditions do not. You should know these and describe the value of staging and how it may help to plan management. If you use words like 'moderate' or 'early' disease, then you should have your mind made up about the answer to the question 'What do you mean by 'moderate?'. Another awful word you may use is 'monitor', as in 'I will monitor disease progression' What do you really mean by that? The actual phrase means virtually nothing. Thus in a case of myocardial infarction it is better to say that you will measure the cardiac enzymes daily rather than 'monitor' them, because that is what the examiner wishes to know.

Another prevalent and annoying response from candidates is to repeat the question. There is almost nothing more infuriating for an examiner than to ask a question and have their words repeated to them. They may feel, subconsciously or otherwise, that the candidate is astonished at the apparent stupidity of the question, which offends them a little, or alternatively that the candidate is deaf. Neither approach is helpful in passing the examination. You may think you never do this, but check with other people and take note of how often other candidates do.

THE ORAL EXAMINATION

The oral examination is designed to assess the breadth of your knowledge, and any topic within the discipline may be tested.

As with the clinical examination, presentation of yourself is important. You will be invited to seat yourself at a table behind which will be two examiners. There may be 'pots' or a slide projector or an X-ray box. You should sit comfortably but should not, for example, cross your legs, as this implies that you are a bit too laid back. Practise sitting down as you would for an interview. Some candidates lean forward in an intimidating manner and may even lean on the table itself. This should also be discouraged as, no matter what people say, the examiners are probably a bit happier with you being intimidated rather than themselves.

The examiners may ask you to comment on your general clinical experience and attempt to make you feel a little more relaxed. They will to some extent be 'feeling you out' to determine the level of questioning they can aim at.

Any one can ask difficult or impossible questions. At the end of each section of cases there is an A–Z of oral-type questions. As in the actual examination these tend to be of two varieties: the question of fact, e.g. 'What are the causes of polyhydramnios?', and the question of management, e.g. 'How would you manage a 21-year-old with acute severe asthma?'.

When you read these questions do not fool yourself by saying 'I read that last night and know it all'. Actually think of how you would answer the question, including the phrases you would use. If you think 'It's OK, I'll read that up later', then think again because you probably won't.

Some of the questions are very straightforward and some are very difficult. Others are strange and even obscure, and some of them are downright bad questions. Answers are provided for all of them, but the management type of question really needs some detail and you should also refer to textbooks. You may also use these as discussion points in your tutorials with clinicians.

The impossible question

Inevitably there will be occasions when you are asked a question which you do not have a clue how to answer. There may be different reasons for this. Let us dispense with the possibility that it might be plain ignorance on your part. One problem is that examiners do sometimes ask questions that are obscure or ambiguous: there can be bad examiners as well as bad candidates. You should have a strategy for dealing with impossible questions: it is important that if you are asked about something you have not even heard of you should say so, in order to move on to something else. If you hum and haw the examiners will assume you are ignorant of this obscure topic, so try to move on rapidly so as to leave them with an impression of knowledge rather than ignorance.

Another type of impossible question is one where you are not certain what the examiner is getting at. This is likely to be a management-type question rather than one of fact. There are three options in this situation. The first is to answer the question as well as you can understand it with as near as possible to a factual answer. Alternatively, if you really do not know what the examiner means, make a simple statement of fact relating to the general topic. With these approaches you will score points with factually correct comments that force the examiner to rephrase the question, hopefully in a better way.

The third option is to make clear that you do not understand the question the way it is phrased. This requires tact, but the other examiner may be grateful to you since he might not see what his colleague is getting at either! This is a final resort but immeasurably better than forcing the examiner to ask the question again because of an embarrassingly prolonged silence. A long silence is time wasted when you should be impressing the examiners.

In answering questions you should try to give all the relevant information you have been asked for. This can be likened to jumping a ravine: with your first answer you want to get right over to the other side. Some candidates leave the exam saying they have answered hundreds of questions, all of them correctly. What they do not realize is that their answers just get them to the crumbly edge at the other side, and every question they answer just keeps them there, without reaching solid ground. In these circumstances you occasionally find examiners of the 'Oh really, Doctor' variety. These are the people who, after you have outlined a course of management or stated a fact, say something like 'Do you really think so?' Sometimes they are trying to make you change your mind, and sometimes will succeed so well that the candidate ends up condemning his or her original opinion. If you are confident that your original answer represented good practice, then you should be able to defend it, although you are at liberty to say that the question addresses a controversial subject.

MEDICINE

HISTORY AND EXAMINATION IN MEDICINE

The essence of history and examination in general medicine is the same as outlined in the introduction, but it does no harm to restate some of the more important points again.

By developing a presentation style with which you are comfortable and familiar, you are less likely to 'go to pieces' in the stressful examination setting. As in the other disciplines when presenting your history and findings, present the key features first. Imagine you are discussing a case on the telephone with a consultant at 2am. He would want to know the crucial information first.

Supplementary information can be added when the stage is set, or when specifically requested, e.g. 'Mr Jones is a 62-year-old gentleman, admitted with an acute myocardial infarction'. You then can go on and discuss the details of the presenting complaint, risk factors etc. The other approach, which is not to be recommended, is to recount the history like a 'whodunnit', leaving the examiner bemused (and probably irritated) until the very last sentence, when you slip in the diagnosis. Focus on the essential features of the history, as this will show the examiners that you know what you are talking about. Look the examiners in the eye as this aids good communication.

Reference to your notes can be useful but do not read them verbatim (remember the short-term memory defect).

Finally, in general medicine in particular, if the patient has a debilitating disease and is likely to need ancillary support, then make sure you have taken a good social history. If the examiners make this a subject of conversation, all you need is some common sense. After taking the history, you will hopefully have a clear idea of the differential diagnosis.

Although a full clinical examination should be carried out, you should seek evidence to establish your diagnosis and be prepared to discuss this. Indeed, many examiners will ask you if your clinical findings are consistent with the patient's history. While performing the examination imagine that someone is going to challenge your diagnosis. You need to be in a position to defend your case. Importantly, whether in the long or short cases, always ask the patient for permission to examine them and make sure you don't inflict pain. It is wise to finish your examination with 5 minutes to spare: this allows you to collect your thoughts and decide how you are going to present the case. You may wish to memorize your opening lines. Some examiners may take you back to the patient and ask you to demonstrate some of your findings (e.g. hyperreflexia). You will impress if you adopt a confident professional approach when returning to the bedside. If you have previously elicited pain when examining a sore joint, for example, it is fair to say that you noted this during your previous examination rather than hurting the patient unnecessarily.

Try to anticipate some likely questions. This may sound obvious, but if you know the answer to the question, say so.

THE CASES

CEREBROVASCULAR DISORDERS ★★★★★

Patients with cerebrovascular disease such as cerebrovascular accident (CVA) or transient ischaemic attack (TIA) are very likely to be included in final exams.

DEFINITIONS

- **Transient ischaemic attack** A focal neurological deficit resulting from cerebral ischaemia which resolves completely within 24 hours.
- **Cerebrovascular accident/stroke** A focal neurological deficit due to a vascular lesion which persists for longer than 24 hours if the patient survives.

HISTORY

The nature of cerebrovascular disease often results in difficulty even taking the history. Distinguish, if you can, whether the patient is acutely confused, dysphasic or dysarthric. It is not enough just to say it was impossible to obtain a history. Say why. If you can obtain a history, then, as with any disease state, obtain an accurate history of the events. Which function was first impaired? How has the deficit worsened or improved? Were there any premonitory symptoms (approximately 25% report a prior TIA)? Was speech or understanding affected? Attention must also be directed to risk factors, e.g. smoking, family history, hypertension, diabetes, obesity and the oral contraceptive pill. Find out how many cigarettes are smoked, whether hypertension has been treated etc. Also establish whether there is evidence of other vascular disease, e.g. myocardial ischaemia or peripheral vascular disease.

EXAMINATION

The clinical diagnosis of a stroke is usually straightforward. Remember, however, that if signs of neurological deficit are persisting, then by definition you cannot diagnose a TIA. General examination should note evidence of hyperlipidaemia (e.g. corneal arcus in the relatively young patient, or xanthelasma), facial asymmetry, gaze paresis or typical hemiplegic posture. You should look for any source of emboli, such as atrial fibrillation or carotid bruits. Measuring the blood pressure is mandatory. You should have examined the fundi as part of the specific neurological work-up, but remember to identify signs of hypertensive retinopathy.

You should systematically examine the central nervous system, including the cranial nerves. Look for evidence of homonymous hemianopia and facial weakness. Power–tone reflexes and sensation should be assessed for all limbs, remembering that all limbs may initially be flaccid in the early stages of an acute stroke. It is unlikely that an acute case will be seen in the clinical finals, but you may well be asked 'What would you expect to have found if you had seen this patient in the acute phase?'

To avoid confusion when describing findings it is often better to refer to left-sided weakness or hemiplegia, rather than right-sided CVA. This is the kind of statement which can start examiners asking about cerebrovascular anatomy and dominant hemispheres etc!

FACTFILE

1. Transient ischaemic attacks (TIA) are an important prognostic event.
2. Within 5 years of a TIA 1 out of 6 patients will have suffered a stroke.
3. Within 5 years of a TIA 1 in 4 will die (usually from heart disease or stroke).
4. Approximately 80% of strokes are thromboembolic, whereas 20% arise from intracranial haemorrhage.
5. Within the first month, mortality from a thromboembolic CVA is less than 25%; approximately 75% with a haemorrhagic CVA will die.
6. Physiotherapy is important in the early stages of a stroke, preventing contractures and improving mobility with the use of walking aids.
7. Frequent turning of the patient will prevent bed sores, a major cause of morbidity.
8. Anticoagulation for atrial fibrillation and treatment of hypertension have been shown in large trials to be beneficial in cerebrovascular disease.

DISCUSSION POINTS

1. This will often address risk factor modification: treatment of hypertension, atrial fibrillation and cessation of smoking etc.
2. Be familiar with early indicators of a poor prognosis after a stroke (e.g. coma, severe hemiplegia, gaze paresis).

CHEST PAIN ★★★★★

Chest pain is one of the most common reasons for acute admission to hospital. It is not surprising that it is also one of the most common conditions encountered in the final examinations. In the exam the most likely causes of chest pain are:

Ischaemic heart disease
1. Angina pectoris ★★★★★
2. Myocardial Infarction ★★★★★

Pleuritic pain
1. Pulmonary thromboembolism ★★★★
2. Pneumothorax ★★★★
3. Oesophageal pain ★★★

DEFINITIONS
- **Angina pectoris** – literally means pain in the chest, assumed to be due to ischaemia of the myocardium.
- **Myocardial infarction** – arises when necrosis of the cardiac muscle occurs.
- **Pneumonia** – inflammation of the lung, usually arising from bacterial or viral infection.
- **Pulmonary embolism** – a condition arising from the passage of thrombus from the systemic veins or, occasionally, the right heart to the pulmonary arteries, resulting in pulmonary infarction and occasionally acute right ventricular failure.
- **Pneumothorax** – air in the pleural space.

HISTORY

The important features of cardiac pain are the relationship to exertion, the radiation to arm, jaw or neck, and the character of the pain, which is classically crushing and central. The use of a clenched fist to describe the pain is highly suggestive of a cardiac origin. Patients who describe a stabbing pain or point with one finger to the source of pain are unlikely to be experiencing myocardial ischaemia. Note typical risk factors of family history, smoking, diabetes, hypertension, previous myocardial infarction and elevated cholesterol.

Pleuritic pain is usually well described by patients. Associated dyspnoea is almost universal. Sputum production, haemoptysis or fever may suggest an infective origin. Coexistent calf pain or predisposing factors for deep venous thrombosis (DVT) should be sought. In women ask about oral contraceptive usage. Although with modern oral contraceptives such cases are unlikely, it is one of the risk factors consultants often ask about.

In young asthenic males with pleuritic pain a pneumothorax is highly likely. A history of chest wall trauma is obviously relevant.

Oesophageal pain is notoriously difficult to differentiate from pain with a cardiac origin. In addition, oesophageal and cardiac pathology often coexist. A history of previous investigation, such as barium meal or upper gastrointestinal endoscopy with definite evidence of hiatus hernia or reflex oesophagitis is worthy of note. Symptoms of 'heartburn' which are worse when bending over or recumbent suggest a possible oesophageal origin, but don't forget that decubitus angina is a recognized phenomenon.

EXAMINATION

Examination in ischaemic heart disease is frequently unhelpful. Look for signs of anaemia or thyrotoxicosis, which may precipitate or worsen the ischaemic symptoms. Xanthelasma or xanthomata should be noted. Occasionally there may be a cardiac murmur of relevance (e.g. aortic stenosis). Evidence of cardiac failure post myocardial infarction is relevant prognostically. In patients with pleuritic chest pain look for asymmetry of chest wall expansion and comment on whether the patient is tachypnoeic or breathless. The presence of fever, anaemia, finger clubbing or emaciation should not be overlooked. Staining of the fingers related to cigarette use is worthy of comment.

If a sputum pot is present you must examine the contents. Look for evidence of deep venous thrombosis.

FACTFILE

1. MI is the most common cause of death in the UK.
2. 20% of patients die within the first 4 hours, most before admission to hospital.
3. The commonest cause of myocardial infarction is thrombus formation on an atherosclerotic plaque in a coronary artery.
4. Very occasionally, myocardial infarction may occur with normal coronary arteries, e.g. embolus, spasm, profound hypotension, aortic stenosis.
5. The following medications have been shown to reduce mortality post myocardial infarction:
   - Aspirin
   - Thrombolytic therapy (e.g. streptokinase)
   - Beta-blockers
   - ACE inhibitors
   - Simvastatin.
6. Pneumothorax may be asymptomatic and small pneumothoraces can be managed conservatively.
7. Larger pneumothoraces will require drainage and, if recurrent, may require pleurodesis.
8. A tension pneumothorax occurs when air accumulates in the pleural space with each inspiration, but cannot escape. This is an emergency and requires immediate treatment.
9. Pneumonia remains a significant cause of mortality, especially in the elderly or debilitated.
10. The most common cause of pneumonia is *Streptococcus pneumoniae* (approximately 50% of cases).
11. The term 'atypical pneumonia' is used to describe pneumonia caused by mycoplasma, influenza A virus, chlamydia and coxiella. This may account for up to 20% of cases.   *(Cont'd)*

12. Rarer causes of pneumonia include chemical causes (e.g. aspiration, radiotherapy).
13. Approximately 50% of cases of pulmonary embolus have evidence of a deep venous thrombosis (DVT).
14. A pulmonary thromboembolus is a common finding at autopsy but is less often diagnosed clinically. Approximately 10% of clinical cases are fatal.
15. The ECG is often unhelpful in the diagnosis of pulmonary thromboembolism.
16. The mainstay is i.v. heparin; larger pulmonary thromboembolism may require thrombolytic therapy or surgical embolectomy.

DISCUSSION POINTS

1. Be prepared to discuss the complications of MI and the role of secondary prevention or risk factor modification.
2. The role of exercise tolerance testing in patients with ischaemic heart disease is important and may be discussed.
3. Be aware of the absolute and relative contraindications to thrombolytic therapy.
4. The management of tension pneumothorax and the conditions associated with pneumothorax (i.e. virtually any respiratory disease) may come up. You must know the principles of the management of the common medical emergencies and be able to describe the practical aspects of management. This includes pneumothorax.
5. Be prepared to discuss the possible causes of a pneumonia not responding to antibiotic therapy, e.g. atypical pneumonia, underlying neoplasm, tuberculosis etc.
6. Which conditions are associated with DVT?

MEDICINE

DIABETES MELLITUS ★★★★★

DEFINITION

A state of hyperglycaemia arising from insufficient or ineffective endogenous insulin.

HISTORY

Important points in the history are symptoms of hyperglycaemia, i.e. polyuria, polydypsia and weight loss. A past medical history of diabetic emergencies should be noted. The presenting feature of diabetes may be one of the complications, e.g. arterial disease, retinopathy, neuropathy, skin infections, renal disease and autonomic neuropathy (diarrhoea, impotence). Establish how long the patient has been diabetic and establish in detail what treatment is currently being used. It is not enough just to say that the patient takes insulin twice daily. Take a dietary history and establish whether blood or urine monitoring is performed at home.

If the patient keeps a diary of blood or urinary monitoring then you may use it (and may even be asked to comment on it by the examiners).

EXAMINATION

This may be directed by the history. You should assess skin condition, insulin injection sites and all pulses. Blood pressure must be recorded. Neurological examination should establish the presence or absence of reflexes and of sensory deficit (light touch and vibration sense). Ideally eye examination should be performed with dilated pupils – this is not likely to have been arranged for your benefit, but do mention that you would prefer that the pupils had been dilated before examination. Remember cataracts are more common in diabetics. If a urine sample is available, test for both glucose and protein.

FACTFILE

1. There are half a million cases in the UK, with probably the same number undiagnosed.
2. The aim of treatment is normoglycaemia without causing hypoglycaemia.
3. Basic dietary points are: take unrefined carbohydrates (potatoes, pasta, cereals) instead of refined carbohydrate (Coca Cola and Mars bars). Encourage dietary fibre and polyunsaturated fats. Alcohol may be taken in moderation (high calorie content).
4. Risk of long-term complications increases as diabetic control worsens.
5. Self-monitoring of urine for glycosuria is not a reliable indicator of blood glucose level. Ideally patients on insulin should perform home blood glucose monitoring and keep a diary of readings.
6. Fundoscopy with dilated pupils should be performed annually.
7. Diabetics should see a chiropodist regularly.
8. When persistent proteinuria is present on dipstick testing (> 150 mg/l) the average patient is only 8–10 years from end-stage renal failure. This progressive failure can be slowed slightly by treating hypertension and improving diabetic control.
9. The cornerstone of treatment is diet – its importance cannot be overemphasized.

DISCUSSION POINTS

1. Know the treatment for diabetic emergencies.
2. Be prepared to discuss different insulin regimens.
3. Further discussions are likely to involve the prevention of complications.
4. Occasionally you may need to discuss the pharmacology of oral hypoglycaemic agents.

MEDICINE

FINGER ON THE PULSE ★★★★★

On at least one occasion during your final examination in medicine you will have to examine and report the pulse. This should be a simple task, but the following points are worthy of note. You should comment on:

- rate
- rhythm
- character
- volume

and whether the vessel wall is palpable or not.

RATE

Give an exact figure, never say approximately. Hopefully you will have counted the pulse accurately, and therefore it is entirely inappropriate to say 'approximately' 78/min. Bradycardia is defined as a heart rate below 60 beats/min. The most likely cause in an examination would be beta-blocker therapy. Other possible causes are a previously athletic individual, or hypothyroid patients. Tachycardia is a heart rate greater than 100 beats/min. Common causes are pyrexia, cardiac failure, exercise, anaemia and anxiety (compare with your own).

RHYTHM

If the rhythm is completely regular, then say that it is sinus rhythm. If the pulse is irregular in rhythm and volume, then the diagnosis is atrial fibrillation. In the long case, record both apical and radial rates. If merely asked to examine the pulse in a short case, you will impress the examiners if you also offer to measure the apical rate. Remember, in atrial fibrillation the rate you report is the ventricular rate, e.g. 'the rhythm is atrial fibrillation, with a poorly controlled ventricular rate of 110 beats/min.'

If the rhythm is basically regular with occasional extra added beats, this is likely to be an ectopic beat.

CHARACTER

If asked to examine the pulse always raise the arm to check for a collapsing pulse, which is indicative of aortic incompetence or, very occasionally, patent ductus arteriosus.

FACTFILE

1. The following are the most common causes of atrial fibrillation:
   - ischaemic heart disease
   - mitral valve disease
   - congestive cardiac failure
   - hypertension
   - alcohol
   - thyrotoxicosis.
2. Approximately 10% of the population over 65 have atrial fibrillation.
3. The risk of embolic stroke is approximately 3–5% per year.
4. 'Lone' AF in the under-60s has a low risk of embolism.

DISCUSSION POINTS

1. This is likely to include the possible causes of atrial fibrillation.
2. Be prepared to discuss the role of anticoagulant therapy in atrial fibrillation.
3. Be prepared to discuss the pharmacological treatment of atrial fibrillation.

HYPERTENSION ★★★★★

Occasionally in the finals you may encounter a patient who has been admitted for investigation and/or treatment of hypertension, or indeed following admission with one of its complications. It is hard to define what is an abnormally high BP, but >160/95 mmHg is commonly regarded as being hypertensive. More than 90% of cases of hypertension have no identified single cause (i.e. essential hypertension). In the exam, however, you are probably more likely to encounter secondary causes of hypertension than you would in routine practice.

Causes of systemic hypertension

1. Essential >90% ★★★★★
2. Secondary causes ★★★
   (a) Renal disease (esp. renovascular)
   (b) Endocrine disorders:
       Cushing's syndrome
       Conn's syndrome
       phaeochromocytoma
       acromegaly
   (c) Coarctation of the aorta ★ (but possible in paediatrics)
   (d) Pregnancy ★ (but very likely in obstetrics)
   (e) Drugs: ★★
       oral contraceptives
       corticosteroids
       antimigraine (ergotamine, sumatriptan)
       erythropoietin
       sympathomimetics (cold and flu remedies).

HISTORY

Enquire how long the patient has been hypertensive and whether they have received treatment. Ask about risk factors such as alcohol, smoking, exercise and diet (including salt and fat). Determine whether there is a previous history of cardiovascular or renal disease. Drug history (including compliance) and family history are noteworthy. Hypertension is usually asymptomatic but at higher levels may occasionally cause headache. If headache is associated with palpitations, tremor, flushing or sweating a phaeochromocytoma should be suspected.

EXAMINATION

In most patients the only sign will be the high BP. Check BP in both arms and, if time allows, recheck after a further 5 minutes. Feel all pulses, especially radial and femorals. Cardiac examination may reveal an apical heave and loud aortic second sound. Listen for abdominal, carotid and femoral bruit. Fundoscopy is essential. Always look for any pointer to a secondary cause, e.g. cushingoid features, acromegaly, enlarged polycystic kidneys.

FACTFILE

1. Management of hypertension must first address lifestyle issues, such as smoking, alcohol intake, weight reduction and exercise.
2. The mortality and morbidity risk increases as BP increases.
3. Secondary hypertension should be considered if age <35, hypokalaemia (not on diuretics) or resistant to therapy.
4. The presence of left ventricular hypertrophy on the ECG represents a significant mortality risk but can regress following improved BP control.
5. 'Routine' investigations should include U+Es (urea and electrolytes), CXR and ECG to assess target organ damage.
6. Poor drug compliance is a recognized problem in hypertensives (because patients experience more symptoms from the drugs than from the disease).
7. Improved BP control has been shown to reduce the incidence of myocardial infarction (MI) and to reduce both incidence and mortality from CVA.

DISCUSSION POINTS

1. This will usually centre on risk factor modification.
2. Be prepared to discuss the pharmacology and side effects of antihypertensive drugs.
3. Why should we bother treating hypertension?
4. What do you consider an abnormally high BP?

CARDIAC MURMURS ★★★★

Murmurs are most often seen as short cases.

Undergraduates usually experience the greatest anxiety and heartache when asked to perform cardiac auscultation. It is important to remember that you are not expected to identify every cardiac lesion, but you should be able to time the murmur, describe where it is best heard and where it radiates to. You are far more likely to impress by performing a thorough, confident examination than by correctly diagnosing a 'full house' of cardiac murmurs using a poor technique. Don't worry about grading the murmur (3/6 etc.): it is more important to give a good description and suggest the most likely lesion. Remember that some murmurs may be heard equally loudly throughout the praecordium (and indeed may radiate widely), so you may be unable to distinguish between, for example, aortic stenosis and mitral regurgitation. If this happens, don't panic. Describe your findings fully and be prepared to admit your uncertainty, offering a logical differential diagnosis.

A few '*ALWAYS*'

1. Always sit the patient at 45°.
2. Always feel the carotid pulse during auscultation.
3. Always roll the patient on to their left side to listen for mitral lesions.
4. Always listen in the neck.

5. Always sit the patient forward and ask them to hold their breath in expiration. Listen for the absence of complete silence during diastole – if aortic incompetence is present you will invariably hear it.
6. Practice is vital: do it often and always follow the same technique until you can perform it automatically, even in the most stressful situations.
7. If you are uncertain whether a murmur is systolic or diastolic remember this moderately insulting but generally fair observation: if the undergraduate can hear it easily it must be systolic!

DYSPNOEA ★★★★

DEFINITION

Dyspnoea is a subjective awareness of difficulty in breathing. The most likely causes in final exam cases will be due to:

- congestive cardiac failure ★★★★★
- chronic obstructive airways disease ★★★★★
- asthma ★★★★★
- pneumonia ★★★★★
- pleural effusion ★★★★
- bronchial carcinoma ★★★★
- pulmonary fibrosis ★★★
- cystic fibrosis ★★★

HISTORY

Try to establish whether the cause of dyspnoea is cardiac or respiratory in origin (or both). Orthopnoea or paroxysmal nocturnal dyspnoea suggests a cardiac cause. A past medical history of myocardial infarction or rheumatic fever is relevant. A detailed smoking history is essential.

Remember the six cardinal symptoms of respiratory disease: cough, sputum, haemoptysis, dyspnoea, wheeze and pain. In a patient with asthma, ask about nocturnal or exertional symptoms. A history of atopy should be sought. Exposure to industrial agents or household pets should be noted.

NB: If you encounter a young patient with finger clubbing, dyspnoea and sputum production in the finals, they will almost certainly have cystic fibrosis. Establish the family history and, if you can, produce a genetic pedigree chart. This should impress.

EXAMINATION

You should be guided by history, but seek evidence of cardio-vascular or respiratory disease. Look for clubbing, finger staining associated with cigarette use, signs of anaemia and weight loss. Comment on respiratory rate and presence of cyanosis. Coexistent eczema in a young person with inter-mittent dyspnoea suggests asthma. Respiratory examination should note the hyperinflated chest of emphysema/chronic obstructive airways disease.

Tracheal deviation is rarely detected but should be sought. Asymmetric chest expansion may reveal underlying lung pathology. The table below gives some indication of findings in patients with the commoner causes of breathlessness.

If any abnormalities are detected, establish whether these are consistent with the patient's history.

Cardiovascular examination should detect cardiomegaly, elevated jugular venous pulse (JVP), cardiac murmurs and basal crepitations which may point to a specific cardiac cause of dyspnoea.

Pathology	CWM	MD	PN	BS	VR
Consolidation	Reduced on affected side	None	Dull	High-pitched Bronchial	Increased
Collapse	Reduced on affected side	Towards lesion	Dull	High-pitched Bronchial	Increased
Pleural effusion	Reduced on affected side	Away from lesion	Stony Dull	Diminished or absent	Reduced or absent
Pneumothorax	Reduced on affected side	Away from lesion	Normal or hyperresonant	Diminished or absent	Reduced or absent

CWM, chest wall movement; MD, mediastinal displacement; PN, percussion note; BS, breath sounds; VR, vocal resonance.

Don't forget to comment on a pleural rub if present. Finally, make sure your findings are consistent, for example don't diagnose a pleural effusion on the basis of a dull percussion note and reduced breath sounds if you have already reported increased vocal resonance.

FACTFILE

1. Asthma is a generalized airways obstruction which, in the early stages at least, is paroxysmal and reversible.
2. The following features suggest a severe attack of asthma:
   (a) use of accessory muscles of respiration
   (b) inability to speak
   (c) severe tachycardia (or worse, bradycardia)
   (d) diminished breath sounds
   (e) cyanosis
   (f) normal or increased $P\text{co}_2$ ($P\text{co}_2$ usually decreases in asthma owing to hyperventilation).
3. Never settle for a diagnosis of 'congestive cardiac failure'. Try to identify the cause, e.g. ischaemic heart disease or valvular heart disease.
4. Staining of the fingers is caused by tar, not nicotine. This seems rather trivial, but may be a source of amusement for the examiner.
5. In chronic bronchitis the most consistent finding is hypertrophy of the mucus-secreting glands of the bronchial tree.
6. Cor pulmonale is right heart failure secondary to chronic lung disease.

DISCUSSION POINTS

1. The management of emergencies such as acute severe asthma and acute pulmonary oedema might well be discussed. As with problems such as acute myocardial infarction, the examiner will wish to know that you are a 'safe' first-line doctor in such emergencies.
2. The difference between a transudate and an exudate, and the causes of each, provides a fund of questions for the examiners and they will expect you to know them.
3. The causes and features of finger clubbing are well worth knowing and can lead to discussion of a variety of problems, from lung disease to inflammatory bowel disease.
4. Be aware of the common causes of occupational lung disease in the UK.
5. Be prepared to discuss the investigation of bronchial carcinoma and assessment for possible surgical treatment.

SKIN DISEASE ★★★★

Dermatology patients are often included in final exams for two reasons:

1. They are usually otherwise well, give a good history and have obvious signs.
2. They are often bored in the dermatology ward and will volunteer for almost anything for a change of scenery for a few hours.

The most likely conditions encountered in the finals are:

- psoriasis ★★★★★
- dermatitis/eczema ★★★★★
- drug-induced reaction ★★★★
- vasculitis ★★★
- malignant melanoma ★★

HISTORY

Determine the extent of the disease (including scalp involvement) and what agents have been in contact with the skin, e.g. domestic, industrial or therapeutic. Also important is to establish the impact of the condition on day-to-day life (for example, application of coal tar). Never forget to take a full drug history. Think of possible underlying disease which may be associated, e.g. eczema and asthma. Precipitating factors such as heat or sunlight should be sought. A family history may be of relevance.

EXAMINATION

As with any clinical examination valuable information can be obtained from the end of the bed. We are often told to use our eyes, but if you have to examine a patient with a dermatological condition you should also use your sense of smell – if the patient smells of coal tar then the diagnosis is psoriasis. Be sure to examine all areas, including the scalp. Look for evidence of excoriation. Be able to describe the distribution and pattern of the disease, e.g. linear, ring lesions. The standard dermatological terminology should be used for lesions, such as macule, papule, vesicle etc.

Note that psoriasis usually affects extensor surfaces, whereas eczema predominates in the flexor aspects. If the diagnosis is psoriasis, look for nail and arthritic changes. The presence of a vasculitic rash should direct you to the possibility of connective tissue diseases.

1. Psoriasis affects approximately 2% of the population.
2. Psoriatic arthropathy occurs in approximately 7% of patients with psoriasis.
3. The presence of arthropathy does not correlate with the extent of skin involvement.
4. Lithium carbonate and beta-blockers are recognized causes of exacerbations of psoriasis.
5. The prognosis in melanoma is related to the depth of the lesion at diagnosis (Breslow thickness).
6. Patch testing may be of value in the investigation of dermatitis, but should only be performed when the original skin disease is in a quiescent phase.
7. Latex allergy appears to be becoming much commoner among healthcare workers.

DISCUSSION POINTS

1. A multitude of drugs can cause skin reactions: be aware of the most common associations. Please note, however, that answering 'Antibiotics' will immediately be followed by 'Which ones?' You should therefore try to be more specific, but if all else fails and you are uncertain which ones, then sulphonamides is usually a good starter for ten.
2. Be prepared to discuss alternatives to coal tar in the treatment of psoriasis.
3. Increasing awareness of the allergens that cause dermatitis makes this a popular topic.

SORE JOINTS ★★★★

Arthritis is inflammation of the joint(s). The main types of arthritis are:

- osteoarthritis (OA) ★★★★★
- rheumatoid arthritis ★★★★★
- infective arthritis ★★
- connective tissue (CT) disorders, e.g. SLE and systemic sclerosis ★★★★
- reactive arthritis ★★★
- ankylosing spondylitis ★★★
- psoriatic arthritis ★★★
- gout ★★★

HISTORY

Establish which joint(s) are most affected, what time of day they are most sore and what degree of disability is present. How does the disability affect the activities of daily living (e.g. dressing, washing etc.)? Is there a past medical history of trauma to the joint, or is there extra-articular involvement (e.g. lungs, eyes)? Is there a family history of similar illness? Is there a history of autoimmune disease?

EXAMINATION

Always ask the patient if the joints are sore before touching them. Look for the cardinal signs of inflammation: heat, swelling, tenderness and redness. Does the patient appear anaemic? The classic rheumatoid changes, if present, should be obvious. Don't forget to look for rheumatoid nodules, a sign of seropositive rheumatoid arthritis. If possible, test the patient's ability to use a pen, cutlery, comb etc. Look for evidence of muscle wasting and extra-articular involvement, e.g. scleritis, vasculitis, rashes (SLE, psoriasis).

FACTFILE

1. A single red, hot joint should be aspirated, looking for infection or crystals, gout or pseudogout.
2. Rheumatoid arthritis is a common illness afflicting approximately 2% of the world population. Because of its systemic nature, rheumatoid disease is an appropriate term.
3. General anaesthesia (with endotracheal intubation) may be complicated in patients with rheumatoid disease because of cervical spine involvement, particularly around the odontoid process.
4. Felty's syndrome is characterized by rheumatoid arthritis, splenomegaly and neutropenia. Recurrent infections are common.
5. The level of erythrocyte sedimentation rate (ESR), C-reactive protein and rheumatoid factor reflects disease activity in rheumatoid disease.
6. In rheumatoid arthritis the disease process can be modified by appropriate treatment, but this is not the case in osteoarthritis.

DISCUSSION POINTS

1. Be prepared to discuss how rheumatoid arthritis may affect the patient's ability to perform everyday tasks, especially personal hygiene.
2. Know which drugs can be used as suppressive agents in the treatment of rheumatoid arthritis, and what the side effects are.
3. Be prepared to discuss the extra-articular features of rheumatoid arthritis and the other connective tissue diseases.

MEDICINE

THE PATIENT WITH WEIGHT LOSS/DEBILITY ★★★★

Patients under investigation for the above symptoms are ideal long cases, which require the candidate to draw out the most likely cause(s) from an extensive list of possibilities.

Weight loss/debility associated with anorexia:

1. Occult malignancy ★★★★★
2. Tuberculosis ★★★★
3. Infective endocarditis ★★★
4. Severe congestive cardiac failure ★★★★
5. Alcoholism ★★★
6. Uraemia ★★★
7. Rheumatoid disease ★★★
8. Neurological disease, e.g. motor neurone disease ★★
9. Dementia (self neglect) ★

Weight loss/debility not associated with anorexia (less common):

1. Diabetes mellitus ★★★★
2. Hyperthyroidism ★★★

HISTORY

Remember that approximately 80% of diagnoses will be made from the history. First, establish whether the patient has lost his or her appetite. This will direct you to the above list(s). Important points in the history would be the presence of altered bowel habit, dysphagia, cough, haemoptysis or dyspnoea. A history of cigarette and alcohol consumption is important. A past medical history of rheumatic fever or ischaemic heart disease should be noted. Also, try to obtain an estimate of the severity of weight loss and over what time period. Many patients will be uncertain of how much weight has been lost, but will be able to tell you if clothes are looser fitting. Women will usually be able to tell if they have 'gone down a size' in clothes.

EXAMINATION

Areas worthy of special attention may be evident from the history. Look for objective evidence of weight loss. Pigmentation (jaundice, uraemia) or lack of it (anaemia), clubbing and lymphadenopathy should be noted. Is there a thyroid mass? Thereafter, each system should be examined in turn. During examination the cardiovascular system should be assessed for new murmurs or evidence of congestive cardiac failure. Respiratory examination may reveal evidence of neoplasia or persistent infection. Abdominal examination may be fruitful, revealing hepatosplenomegaly (haematological malignancy), right iliac fossa mass (Crohn's disease) or ascites. Do not perform a rectal examination, but make sure you tell the examiners that you would wish to.

FACTFILE

1. A massively enlarged spleen will almost certainly be due to chronic myeloid leukaemia or myelofibrosis. (Kala azar and malaria are uncommon in western Europe, so don't offer either as your first cause of splenomegaly.)
2. Tuberculosis is on the increase again and drug resistance is becoming a problem.
3. A patient with general malaise and a predisposing cardiac abnormality should be treated as having infective endocarditis until proved otherwise.
4. Morbidity rates for alcohol consumption follow a J-shaped, curve i.e. morbidity is higher among those with no alcohol use than in moderate drinkers. Heavier consumption is associated with a considerable increase in morbidity.

DISCUSSION POINTS

1. Be prepared to discuss the investigation of patients with unexplained weight loss and debility. Try to be logical and don't offer the 'smokescreen' list of all possible investigations. Remember, a lot of information can be gained from the simple tests, e.g. full blood count (FBC), chest X-ray, liver function tests and blood cultures. Computed tomography (CT) and magnetic resonance imaging (MRI) scans are never your first investigation of choice.
2. Why might the incidence of tuberculosis be on the increase and why might drug resistance occur?
3. In a patient with infective endocarditis, what are the possible sources of infection?

BLACKOUTS ★★★

No strict definition for blackouts can be made. Indeed, patients will have very different ideas of what a blackout is. A history of 'blackouts' is a very common presenting disorder, and your ability to obtain a good history will be crucial.

CAUSES OF BLACKOUTS

Neurological

1. Epilepsy ★★★★★
2. Vertebrobasilar ischaemia ★★★★★
3. Ménière's disease ★

Cardiac

1. Myocardial infarction ★★★★
2. Aortic stenosis ★★★★

3. Arrythmias ★★★★
4. Postural hypotension ★★★★★
5. Stokes–Adams attacks ★★★★

Drug-induced
1. Antihypertensives ★★★
2. Glyceryl trinitrate ★★
3. Tricyclic antidepressants ★
4. L-dopa ★
5. Insulin/oral hypoglycaemics ★

HISTORY

Establish what the patient means by a 'blackout' and the circumstances in which they occur (e.g. after coughing or micturition). How frequent are they and how long do they last? How do they feel afterwards (e.g. post-ictal)? Do they lose consciousness? Have eye-witnesses told the patient what they have seen? Is there a warning to the attack? Are there other features? Also, enquire about significant past medical history and drug history. Ensure that the history includes non-prescription drugs, or even those 'borrowed from a friend with the same problem'.

EXAMINATION

Examination may be unhelpful, but cardiac and neurological examinations may reveal the cause. Direct your examination to identifying the likeliest cause based upon history and risk factors. In particular listen for carotid bruit and check lying and standing blood pressures.

FACTFILE

1. **Painless myocardial infarction is a recognized cause of blackouts in the elderly, diabetic or hypertensive patient.**
2. **Once symptoms arise from aortic stenosis the prognosis is poor: investigation with a view to valve replacement is therefore indicated.**
3. **An epileptic seizure can be defined as a transient abnormal event, triggered by abnormal electrical activity of cerebral neurones.**
4. **A diagnosis of epilepsy has major social implications (e.g. work, driving, leisure pursuits).**
5. **Non-compliance is a cause of apparently uncontrolled epilepsy and should be remembered when considering these patients.**

DISCUSSION POINTS

1. Know the definition of status epilepticus.
2. What are the driving regulations for patients with a diagnosis of epilepsy?
3. Know the side effects of the commoner anticonvulsant drugs.
4. In cases of young women you may discuss the risk of fetal abnormality with epilepsy with and without anticonvulsants.

DEMENTIA ★★★

DEFINITION

A progressive generalized failure of higher cerebral function.

Patients with dementia may occasionally be used in the exam if 'quality' cases are sparse in the medical wards (as is not infrequently the case). You should know how to perform abbreviated mental testing as follows.

More than four of the following questions incorrect suggests a diagnosis of dementia:

1. Age
2. Time (to nearest hour)
3. Address for recall at end of test, e.g. 26 Smith Street
4. Year
5. Name of this place
6. Recognition of two persons (doctor, nurse etc.)
7. Date of birth
8. Year of the first world war
9. Name of the Prime Minister (make sure you know yourself)
10. Count backwards from 20 to 1.

FACTFILE

1. You may need to make special allowance on question 9: the number of patients who answer that Margaret Thatcher is Prime Minister is amazing. The number of people with no intellectual deficit who cannot remember the name of her successor appears not to be so surprising.

2. If you are asked to perform abbreviated mental testing, make a point of inspecting for obvious causes of impaired mental function, e.g. cerebrovascular disease, hypothyroidism or chronic liver disease.

DISCUSSION POINT

This will centre on the causes of dementia which are treatable. Know some of these causes in case you are asked to discuss them in detail.

DIARRHOEA/CHANGE IN BOWEL HABIT ★★★

Diarrhoea can be defined as an increase in stool weight and/or frequency, but patients may interpret this symptom differently. Change in bowel habit may be seen in either medicine or surgery. Surgical aspects will be discussed later and the causes of diarrhoea are legion, but in the exam you are most likely to encounter:

- inflammatory bowel disease ★★★★★
- colonic neoplasm ★★★★ (but likelier in surgical finals)
- diverticular disease ★★★★
- malabsorption ★★★

Infective, endocrine and drug-induced diarrhoea should not be overlooked, but are unlikely in the exam. Irritable bowel syndrome is also common, but equally unlikely in the medical finals.

HISTORY

Identify what the patient means by diarrhoea or a change in bowel habit. Determine bowel frequency, a description of the stool and whether blood is present. Steatorrhoea suggests malabsorption. Anorexia and weight loss suggest a possible neoplasm. Ask about tenesmus. An acute onset of symptoms points more to an infective cause or dietary indiscretion.

If symptoms are chronic with a relapsing/remitting course, inflammatory bowel disease should be considered. The major symptoms of Crohn's disease are diarrhoea, abdominal pain and weight loss. The major symptom in ulcerative colitis is diarrhoea with mucus and blood, and only occasionally with abdominal pain. Systemic features of malaise, lethargy and anorexia are common in both ulcerative colitis and Crohn's disease. In severe exacerbations nocturnal diarrhoea, urgency and incontinence may occur. Manifestations of inflammatory bowel disease outside the bowel, such as arthritis, should be sought.

EXAMINATION

Look for evidence of weight loss and anaemia. Aphthous ulceration of the mouth is commonly seen in inflammatory bowel disease. Abdominal examination may be unhelpful, but a right iliac fossa mass and fistulae may be seen in Crohn's disease. Look for evidence of extra-gastrointestinal features such as arthritis, iritis etc.

Although you should not perform a rectal examination, the examiners will expect you to acknowledge this as a crucial aspect of investigation. Fortunately stool samples are not usually provided for inspection!

MEDICINE

FACTFILE

1. Crohn's disease is a chronic inflammatory disorder which may affect any part of the gastrointestinal tract, from mouth to anus. Dentists not infrequently make the diagnosis (while examining the mouth!!).

2. The following features suggest a severe attack of ulcerative colitis:
   - Stool frequency >6 stools per day with blood
   - Fever (>37.5°C)
   - Tachycardia
   - ESR >30 mm/h
   - Anaemia – haemoglobin <10 g/dl
   - Albumin <30 g/l.

3. Even in patients with known inflammatory bowel disease, never overlook the possibility of superimposed infection, especially if unresponsive to conventional therapy. Stool culture (including *clostridium dificile*) should always be performed.

4. Patients with ulcerative colitis and Crohn's disease with colonic involvement should take regular 5-ASA-containing compounds (e.g. mesalazine).

5. Coeliac disease is associated with an increased incidence of small bowel lymphoma and carcinoma of the small bowel and oesophagus.

6. In 'unresponsive' coeliac disease always suspect dietary non-compliance.

DISCUSSION POINTS

1. Be prepared to discuss the differences (and similarities) between ulcerative colitis and Crohn's disease.
2. What are the complications of ulcerative colitis (or Crohn's disease)?

3. When might surgery be indicated in inflammatory bowel disease?
4. What are the histological features of coeliac disease?
5. Know the major causes of infective diarrhoea.
6. Know the staging of colonic cancer and the frequency in patients with long-standing ulcerative colitis.

JAUNDICE (medical aspects) ★★★

DEFINITION

Yellow staining of the body tissue secondary to excess circulating bilirubin, usually considered as 40 µmol/l or more.

Classification:
   Prehepatic (haemolytic)
   Hepatic
   Post-hepatic (obstructive)

You may encounter a jaundiced patient in either the medical or surgical final exams. This can be categorized in different ways and it is worth learning a classification system. You may also classify jaundice as conjugated hyperbilirubinaemia or unconjugated hyperbilirubinaemia.

For the purposes of final examinations the following causes should be considered:

- Viral hepatitis ★★★★
- Cirrhosis ★★★★★
- Hepatic malignancy (usually metastatic) ★★★★★
- Gallstones ★ in a medical exam
- Carcinoma of pancreas ★ in a medical exam
- Carcinoma of bile duct ★ in a medical exam
- Drugs (cholestatic or toxic, **NB** paracetamol) ★★★
- Haemolytic (e.g. haemoglobinopathy) ★★
- Congenital hyperbilirubinaemias, e.g. Gilbert's disease) ★★

HISTORY

Determine the duration of illness and whether progressive or not. Bear in mind the age of the patient. Older people with weight loss are likely to have malignancy, whereas young patients are more likely to have hepatitis. Pruritis, stool and urine colour will suggest if there is an obstructive component to the jaundice. An infective cause is suggested by a recent community or family outbreak or recent travel abroad (hepatitis A). Intravenous drug abuse, tattoos, homosexuality or recent transfusion may lead to hepatitis B or C. Farm and sewage workers and others who participate in water sports may contract leptospirosis. Ask about alcohol ingestion and any medication. Women with jaundice and pruritis may have primary biliary cirrhosis. A family history of recurrent jaundice suggests Gilbert's syndrome in Caucasians or haemoglobinopathy in Asians or Africans.

Abdominal pain may be secondary to gallstones and is an important symptom. Obstructive jaundice is more likely to be met as a surgical case and will be discussed elsewhere. Nevertheless, the examiners may well wish to discuss surgical causes of jaundice and you should be prepared for this.

EXAMINATION

Look for the signs of chronic liver disease (spider naevi, palmar erythema, flapping tremor, leuconychia etc.). If hepatomegaly is detected, describe the features (i.e. smooth, firm, regular, irregular, pulsatile etc.). A knobbly, irregular liver suggests metastases. Splenomegaly is usually taken as evidence of portal hypertension. Look for ascites, which is common in cirrhosis. If urine is available, test it.

FACTFILE

1. Chronic hepatitis is defined as any hepatitis lasting 6 months or longer.

2. Cirrhosis is a histological diagnosis: it can be defined as a condition involving the entire liver, with necrosis of hepatocytes followed by fibrosis and nodule formation. These changes are irreversible.

3. Approximately two-thirds of patients with cirrhosis will develop gastro-oesophageal varices, of which approximately one-third will bleed.

4. The following features are poor prognostic indicators in cirrhosis:
   - hypoalbuminaemia
   - hyponatraemia
   - coagulopathy
   - ascites
   - persistent jaundice
   - continued alcohol ingestion
   - neuropsychiatric complications.

5. Primary biliary cirrhosis is a chronic disorder of unknown aetiology, characterized by progressive destruction of the bile ducts. No specific therapy is of proven benefit. Once the serum bilirubin reaches 100 mmol/l liver transplantation is indicated.

6. Hepatocellular carcinoma is a primary hepatic malignancy which is associated with a raised alpha-fetoprotein. Approximately 80% of cases occur in cirrhotic livers.

7. The common causes of hepatomegaly in the adult are:
   - cirrhosis (in later stages of this condition the liver is not palpable)
   - fatty infiltration
   - congestive cardiac failure
   - metastatic cancer
   - hepatitis
   - hepatoma
   - haematological, e.g. leukaemia.

MEDICINE

DISCUSSION POINTS

1. Be able to recognise a cholestatic or hepatocellular picture when shown abnormal liver function tests (LFTs).
2. Have a structured scheme for the investigation of jaundice.
3. What is the cause of pruritis in obstructive jaundice?
4. Know how to treat hepatic encephalopathy and what the precipitating factors might have been.
5. Which malignancies commonly metastasize to the liver?
6. Hepatotoxicity is a recognized complication of many drugs. Which ones?
7. Know the anatomical landmarks of the spleen and how to distinguish it from the left kidney.

NEUROLOGICAL PATIENTS (excluding 'blackouts') ★★★

The most likely neurological conditions you will encounter in the finals are:

- cerebrovascular disease (as discussed previously) ★★★★★
- multiple sclerosis ★★★★
- Parkinson's disease ★★★★
- motor neurone disease ★★★
- epilepsy ★★★★

DEFINITIONS

- **Multiple sclerosis** is a disease of unknown cause characterized by multiple areas of demyelination in the brain and spinal cord. These are disseminated in both time and place.

- **Parkinson's disease** is a progressive degenerative disorder of the extrapyramidal system, characterized by akinesia, rigidity and tremor.
- **Motor neurone disease** is characterized by progressive degeneration of motor neurones in the spinal cord, cranial nerves and cortex.

HISTORY

Patients will usually know the diagnosis and tell you themselves what is wrong. Ascertain whether symptoms have been gradually worsening or arisen acutely. Which functions have been particularly affected (e.g. optic neuritis in multiple sclerosis (MS), swallowing in motor neuron disease)? How is the gait affected? Does the patient 'freeze'? The presence of sensory symptoms excludes a diagnosis of motor neurone disease. As always, find out what impact the disease has had on everyday life. Drug history may be relevant (parkinsonism, cerebellar dysfunction).

EXAMINATION

Important points may be observed during history taking (e.g. cerebellar speech in multiple sclerosis, or the expressionless face of Parkinson's disease). Is there a pill-rolling or intention tremor? Full central nervous system examination should be performed but pay particular attention to those functions the patient finds difficult. Observe the patient walking. Is there a festinant gait, foot drop or cerebellar or spastic ataxia? If you suspect motor neurone disease look for evidence of bulbar dysfunction.

FACTFILE

1. Multiple (disseminated) sclerosis cannot be diagnosed after a single isolated symptom. The lesions, and therefore associated symptoms and signs, must be disseminated in both time and place.
2. Like many diseases, multiple sclerosis may be relapsing and remitting, or may be chronically progressive.
3. MRI scans can now detect areas of demyelination.
4. Evidence that Parkinson's disease may have an environmental aetiology is suggested by the finding that certain experimental agents produce a syndrome indistinguishable from Parkinson's disease in humans and primates.
5. Motor neurone disease has no known cause or treatment. Survival for more than 3 years is rare.

DISCUSSION POINTS

1. How does multiple sclerosis commonly present, what are the favourable prognostic features and what benefits do corticosteroids confer?
2. Be prepared to discuss which agents cause drug-induced parkinsonism and the side-effects of L-dopa therapy.
3. Know the patterns of motor neurone disease.

THYROID PATIENTS (medical aspects) ★★★

Thyroid disorders are very common and increase with age. The diagnosis of thyroid dysfunction is biochemical, but careful history and examination may point to the diagnosis. Remember, however, that only rarely will the classic picture of thyroid disease be present.

HISTORY

Any symptoms of hypo- or hyperthyroidism should be noted. Take a detailed history of past thyroid surgery or radio-iodine treatment.

Drug history is important (e.g. thyroxine, amiodarone, lithium, carbimazole). Ask about a family history of thyroid and other autoimmune disorders.

EXAMINATION

Examination of the neck and thyroid gland itself is discussed in detail in the surgical section of this book. On inspection look for evidence of a goitre, hair loss, tremor, exophthalmos or lid lag. Myxoedema may be present, i.e. subcutaneous mucopolysaccharide accumulation. Are the palms sweaty and is there a tachycardia or atrial fibrillation? Remember to check for slowly relaxing reflexes. Remember to listen for a thyroid bruit and check for retrosternal extension (inability to palpate the lower margin of the gland).

FACTFILE

1. Radioiodine treatment is safe and appropriate in nearly all types of hyperthyroidism, especially in the elderly, but is contraindicated in children, pregnant women and breastfeeding mothers.

2. The main indications for surgery are a large goitre, failed medical treatment, toxic nodular goitre or patient preference.

3. All patients treated with radioiodine or surgery should have yearly checks of thyroid function.

4. Thyroxine treatment should be initiated cautiously in patients with ischaemic heart disease, as the resulting increase in metabolic rate can precipitate acute myocardial infarction or sudden death.

5. Routine screening of the healthy adult population is not justified.

DISCUSSION POINTS

1. Discussion will usually centre on the treatment of hypo- or hyperthyroidism.
2. What are the complications of thyroid surgery?
3. Be prepared to discuss other autoimmune conditions.

ANAEMIC PATIENTS ★★

DEFINITION

Anaemia is present when there is a decrease in the haemoglobin level below the reference range for the age and sex of the individual.

HISTORY

Remember that anaemia is *not* a diagnosis (*cf.* heart failure): a cause must be found. First establish whether there have been symptoms of anaemia or worsening of any underlying disease, such as angina or intermittent claudication. Remember that the patient may have become anaemic gradually and therefore may be asymptomatic. Ask if they have been anaemic before and how it was treated. Pursue any history of blood loss (gastrointestinal, menstrual) or altered bowel habit. A dietary history is essential. Is there any suggestion of malabsorption?

Drug history should be noted (e.g. NSAIDs or cytotoxics). Past medical history will identify conditions associated with 'anaemia of chronic disease'. If the patient is non-Caucasian think of inherited haemoglobinopathies.

CAUSES OF ANAEMIA

1. Hypochromic microcytic – Fe deficiency ★★★★★
2. Normochromic normocytic – anaemia of chronic disease ★★★
3. Macrocytic – B_{12}/folate deficiency ★★★
4. Aplastic anaemia – congenital ★
   – acquired (idiopathic, drugs, radiation, infections) ★★★
5. Marrow invasion – e.g. lymphoma, leukaemia, secondary carcinoma ★★★
6. Haemolytic – hereditary: ★★
   haemoglobinopathy
   cell membrane defects
   enzyme defects
   – acquired:
   autoimmune
   non-autoimmune

EXAMINATION

Check the conjunctivae and palmar creases. Cardiovascular examination may reveal tachycardia, hypotension (actively bleeding patients are unlikely to be exam subjects) or evidence of cardiac failure. Is the patient jaundiced (haemolysis)? Examine carefully for lymphadenopathy, hepatosplenomegaly and abdominal masses. Signs of chronic liver disease are noteworthy (?varices, pancytopenia). Inform the examiner that you would wish to perform a rectal examination and check for faecal occult blood.

INVESTIGATION

The first line of investigation should be a full blood count and film. Thereafter think of anaemia as microcytic, normocytic or macrocytic. Iron-deficiency anaemia indicates the need for gastrointestinal investigation. If macrocytic check B_{12} and folate (also thyroid function tests). In older patients with a low B_{12} a Schilling test is indicated. Investigation and treatment of normochromic normocytic anaemia will be that of the underlying disorder. If haemolysis is present there will be an increased bilirubin and reticulocyte count, with decreased haptoglobins.

FACTFILE

1. Iron is present in meat, liver, eggs, milk and green vegetables.
2. Vitamin B_{12} is found in meat, fish, eggs and milk but not in plants.
3. Dietary folate is usually obtained from green vegetables and offal products.
4. Pernicious anaemia (PA) is associated with gastric atrophy and increased risk of gastric carcinoma.
5. PA must be distinguished from other causes of B_{12} deficiency, such as a vegan diet, terminal ileal disease or bacterial overgrowth in the small bowel.
6. Blood transfusion is rarely required in PA and may precipitate cardiac failure.
7. Pancytopenia (anaemia, leucopenia and thrombocytopenia) suggests marrow failure and examination of the marrow is required.

DISCUSSION POINTS

1. Be prepared to discuss how you would manage a patient with iron-deficiency anaemia.
2. What is hypovolaemic shock and how would you treat it?
3. What are the causes of upper gastrointestinal blood loss?
4. Why are vegans prone to vitamin B_{12} deficiency?
5. Describe the Schilling test procedure.

HEADACHE ★★

Patients complaining of headache frequently present to outpatient clinics or indeed as emergencies. The commonest cause of headache is tension, but you should be aware of the salient features of other types of headache. A detailed history is essential in establishing the correct diagnosis. Determine the exact location and character of the pain, associated features (e.g. photophobia or vomiting), precipitating factors (e.g. chocolate, cheese, shaving) and periodicity. Important points in the history are summarized below:

- Sudden onset of occipital pain with neck stiffness – subarachnoid haemorrhage ★★★
- Unilateral throbbing pain, photophobia and preceding visual aura – migraine ★★
- Shooting 'electric shock' facial pain – trigeminal neuralgia ★★
- Temporal headache, age >50 +/– visual upset – temporal arteritis ★★★
- Worst in the morning with vomiting and/or neurological signs – raised intracranial pressure ★★★
- Intermittent with nasal stuffiness and watery eyes – cluster headache ★★
- Headache with neck stiffness and pyrexia – meningitis ★★★

Remember other possible sources of pathology, such as sinuses, eyes, ears, temporomandibular arthritis and toothache.

Remember that it is unlikely you will be presented with an acute case such as meningitis or subarachnoid haemorrhage, but you will be asked how you might identify the clinical features of such conditions.

EXAMINATION

This may be directed by features in the history. General inspection will reveal any suggestion of weight loss. Photophobia will be obvious. Palpate the temporal arteries and check pulse and BP. Fundoscopy is essential and look for ocular palsies. Although they are unlikely to be present, do check for neck stiffness and Kernig's sign. A full neurological examination should be performed.

FACTFILE

1. Migraine is the most common neurological complaint.
2. Remember the law of thirds in subarachnoid haemorrhage: one-third die, one-third rebleed and one-third survive.
3. A normal CT scan does not exclude a subarachnoid haemorrhage: examination of the CSF is required.
4. Subarachnoid haemorrhage accounts for 10% of cerebrovascular disease.
5. Saccular 'berry' aneurysms account for 70% of subarachnoid haemorrhage.
6. Nimodipine, a calcium channel blocker, has been shown to reduce mortality in subarachnoid haemorrhage.
7. Untreated, 25% of cases of temporal arteritis will result in visual loss due to inflammation of ciliary or central retinal arteries.

DISCUSSION POINTS

1. Be prepared to discuss poor prognostic features in subarachnoid haemorrhage (e.g. age >65, coma, neurological deficit).
2. How would you confirm the diagnosis of subarachnoid haemorrhage and how would you proceed with management?

3. Which individuals are prone to subdural haematoma?
4. Discuss the management of migraine, i.e. avoidance of triggers, prophylaxis and treatment of the acute attack.
5. Which organisms may cause meningitis?

RENAL FAILURE (medical aspects) ★★

DEFINITION

A reduction in renal function with a consequent rise in blood urea and serum creatinine. Acute renal failure develops over a few weeks or days, whereas chronic renal failure develops over months or years. It is unlikely that you will be presented with a patient in acute renal failure.

CAUSES OF CHRONIC RENAL FAILURE

- Glomerulonephritis ★★★★★
- Pyelonephritis/tubulointerstitial nephritis ★★★★★
- Diabetes mellitus ★★★★★
- Hypertension ★★★★
- Calculi ★★★
- Polycystic kidneys ★★★
- Connective tissue diseases ★★★
- Myeloma ★★
- Drugs (e.g. ACE inhibitors, non-steroidal anti-inflammatory drugs, gentamicin) ★★★

HISTORY

This should aim to determine whether the cause of renal failure is likely to be prerenal, renal or postrenal. Are there any predisposing factors to dehydration (e.g. diuretics, diarrhoea or vomiting)? Renal causes may be alluded to if there has been a previous history of renal problems or if there is systemic disease such as diabetes or systemic vasculitis. An accurate drug history is essential. Postrenal causes might be suggested by a history of prostatism or of cancer. Previous urinary calculi may be important, as may a history of abdominal or pelvic surgery. Always remember to document whether there are any symptoms of renal failure, such as nausea, anorexia, vomiting, fluid retention or hypertension. Ask if there has been dysuria, polyuria, haematuria or oliguria. If the patient is on dialysis find out the exact details of this and what impact it has on daily life. Finally, since adult polycystic kidney disease is an autosomal dominant condition, the family history is important.

EXAMINATION

Initially make an assessment of hydration. Dehydration is suggested by reduced tissue turgor, low JVP and a dry-looking tongue. Check the blood pressure for postural drop or hypertension. Fluid overload is likely if there is oedema, a raised JVP or pulmonary oedema. General inspection will reveal pallor or the characteristic lemon-yellow tinge. A vasculitic rash or evidence of pruritis may be apparent. Abdominal examination should document whether there is loin tenderness (tubulonephritis) or renal enlargement (polycystic kidneys) or a palpable bladder (prostate or pelvic pathology). Inform the examiners of the necessity to perform a rectal examination. *Never* forget to perform urinalysis if a sample is present. Note the presence of an AV fistula.

DISCUSSION POINTS

1. Be prepared to discuss the clinical assessment of a patient's fluid balance and know about central venous pressure monitoring.

2. Know the common causes of renal failure requiring dialysis.
3. What are the advantages and disadvantages of haemodialysis and peritoneal dialysis?
4. What are the problems associated with renal transplantation?
5. Other than fluid balance, what regulatory functions does the kidney perform?

FACTFILE

1. Dialysis should be considered when K+ >6 mmol/l, urea >40, fluid overload, HCO <l2 and creatinine >500 μmol/l.

2. Continuous ambulatory peritoneal dialysis (CAPD) is easy to teach, less expensive in the short term, can be performed easily, allows holidays and is less time-consuming. Disadvantages include peritonism (50% in 2 years need to discontinue CAPD), weight gain, hernias and pancreatitis.

3. Haemodialysis is more time-consuming, requiring time off work etc. Haemorrhage, hepatitis, sepsis and cerebral oedema are recognized complications of haemodialysis. Roughly 50% of haemodialysis patients in the UK have home haemodialysis, which alleviates some of these problems, but obviously this has cost implications.

4. Most patients require 12–21 hours of dialysis per week in two or three sessions.

5. Human recombinant erythropoeitin (EPO) is useful in the treatment of anaemia in chronic renal failure. Side effects include hypertension, clotting problems and convulsions.

AN A–Z IN MEDICINE

QUESTIONS

ALCOHOL

A1 What conditions are associated with excess alcohol ingestion?

AMYLOIDOSIS

A2 What conditions predispose to amyloid deposition?

ANAEMIA

A3 How would you approach the investigation of a 60-year-old patient with a haemoglobin of 6 g/dl?

ASTHMA

A4 How would you manage an acute asthma attack?

A5 Why might the incidence of asthma be on the increase?

ATRIAL FIBRILLATION

A6 Should all patients with atrial fibrillation be anticoagulated?

BENCE-JONES PROTEINS

B1 What are Bence-Jones proteins?

BRAIN DEATH

B2 What criteria should be recognized for the diagnosis of brain death?

CARDIAC ENZYMES

C1 What is the time pattern of cardiac enzyme rise in acute myocardial infarction?

CEREBELLUM

C2 What are the causes of cerebellar dysfunction?

CIGARETTES

C3 What disease states are associated with cigarette smoking?

CYSTIC FIBROSIS

C4   What is the pattern of inheritance of cystic fibrosis?

DIABETES

D1   Patients often say they have 'mild' diabetes. Is there such a form of diabetes?

D2   How would you manage a case of diabetic ketoacidosis?

DIGOXIN

D3   What are the side effects of digoxin?

DUODENAL ULCER

D4   How would you investigate and treat a patient with suspected duodenal ulcer?

D5   Is duodenal ulcer an infective disorder?

ECG

E1   Where would you position the leads for a standard 12-lead ECG?

E2   What ECG findings might be present following acute pulmonary embolism?

EISENMENGER'S SYNDROME

E3   What is Eisenmenger's syndrome?

ESR

E4   What is the ESR and is it of value?

FARMER'S LUNG

F1   What is the cause of farmer's lung?

FINGER CLUBBING

F2   What are the features of finger clubbing?

FUNGUS

F3   Which patients are most prone to fungal infections?

GAIT

G1   What abnormal gaits may be recognized while walking down the High Street?

GLASGOW COMA SCALE

G2   What is the Glasgow Coma Scale?

GOUT

G3   What is gout and how would you treat it?

GYNAECOMASTIA

G4   What are the causes of gynaecomastia?

HAEMATEMESIS

H1   What are the possible causes of haematemesis?

HEBERDEN'S NODES

H2   What are Heberden's nodes?

HYPOGLYCAEMIA

H3   How might hypoglycaemia present?

INTRACRANIAL PRESSURE

I1   What signs may be present in rising intracranial pressure?

IRRITABLE BOWEL SYNDROME

I2   What are the features of irritable bowel syndrome?

JACKSONIAN EPILEPSY

J1   What is Jacksonian epilepsy?

JANEWAY LESIONS

J2   What are janeway lesions?

JAUNDICE

J3   What is jaundice and how would you classify it?

JUGULAR VENOUS PULSE

J4   How do you distinguish jugular venous pulsation from arterial?

KIDNEYS

K1   How might a patient with polycystic kidneys present?

KOEBNER PHENOMENON

K2   What is the Koebner phenomenon?

LACUNAR INFARCTION

L1   What is a lacunar infarct?

LEGIONNAIRES' DISEASE

L2   What features may suggest a diagnosis of legionnaires' disease?

L3   Why is legionnaires' disease so called?

LIPIDS

L4   Is lipid-lowering therapy of any benefit?

L5   Should all patients with an elevated cholesterol be treated with lipid-lowering therapy?

MACROCYTIC ANAEMIA

M1   Name some causes of a macrocytic anaemia.

MALIGNANT MELANOMA

M2   How might we reduce mortality from malignant melanoma?

MENINGITIS

M3   What are the symptoms and common causes of meningitis?

MIGRAINE

M4   What drugs are useful in the treatment of migraine?

MYELOMA

M5   What are the diagnostic features of multiple myeloma?

NEPHROTIC SYNDROME

N1   What are the features of nephrotic syndrome? Name some causes.

NON-STEROIDAL ANTI-INFLAMMATORY DRUGS (NSAIDS)

N2   NSAIDs are very commonly used (and abused) drugs. What are their side effects?

OPPORTUNISTIC INFECTION

O1   How would you define opportunistic infection?

OSTEOPOROSIS

O2   Who might suffer from osteoporosis?

PANCYTOPENIA

P1   Name some causes of pancytopenia.

PARACETAMOL POISONING

P2   What are the dangers of paracetamol poisoning?

P3   How would you manage a case of paracetamol poisoning?

PLEURAL EFFUSION

P4   List some causes of pleural effusion.

PLUMMER–VINSON (PATERSON–BROWN–KELLY) SYNDROME

P5   What is Plummer–Vinson syndrome?

PULMONARY OEDEMA

P6   Describe the management of acute pulmonary oedema.

PUO (PYREXIA OF UNKNOWN ORIGIN)

P7   What conditions may present as PUO?

QT INTERVAL

Q1   What are the causes of a long QT interval?

RAYNAUD'S PHENOMENON

R1   How would you define Raynaud's phenomenon and what are the aetiological factors?

REITER'S SYNDROME

R2   What is Reiter's syndrome?

RHEUMATOID ARTHRITIS

R3   What are the features that distinguish rheumatoid arthritis from osteoarthritis?

SARCOIDOSIS

S1 What is sarcoidosis and what features may be seen on chest X-ray?

SCREENING

S2 A number of screening tests have been advocated (e.g. cholesterol, blood pressure). What criteria would the ideal screening test fulfil?

SHOCK

S3 Can you define shock, and discuss some of the causes (**NB**: this does not mean the type beloved by the media, which responds to a cup of tea in the Accident & Emergency Department!).

STEROIDS

S4 What are the side effects of corticosteroid therapy?

STREPTOKINASE

S5 What are the side effects of streptokinase and when might its administration be contraindicated?

THYROTOXICOSIS

T1 What are the typical symptoms in thyrotoxicosis?

TRANSPLANTATION

T2 How might we increase the number of donor organs available?

TRIGEMINAL NEURALGIA

T3 What are the classic features of trigeminal neuralgia and how might it be treated?

TUBERCULOSIS

T4 Which organs are affected by tuberculosis?
T5 Which patients are particularly prone to such infection?

ULCERATIVE COLITIS

U1 What are the complications of ulcerative colitis?

U2   What features would suggest a poorer prognosis?

ULTRASOUND

U3   In what diseases may ultrasound information be of value?

VIRAL INFECTION

V1   What is the role of zidovudine in HIV infection?

VITAMINS

V2   What symptoms and signs may arise from vitamin deficiencies?

WERNICKE'S ENCEPHALOPATHY

W1   What is Wernicke's encephalopathy?

WILSON'S DISEASE

W2   What do you know about Wilson's disease?

X-CHROMOSOME

X1   Can you name some X-linked disorders?

X-RAY

X2   What are the possible abnormalities in a chest X-ray which at first sight appear normal and might be missed on initial inspection?

ZOLLINGER—ELLISON SYNDROME

Z1   What do you know about Zollinger—Ellison syndrome?

ANSWERS

A1   *Cardiac:* Hypertension, atrial fibrillation, cardiomyopathy;

Gastrointestinal: Gastritis, varices, oesophageal carcinoma, pancreatitis, cirrhosis;

Neurological: Cerebral atrophy, subdural haematoma, epilepsy, neuropathy, head injury, Wernicke–Korsakoff syndrome;

Bone: Osteoporosis, fractures;

Haematology: Marrow suppression;

A2   Rheumatoid arthritis, bronchiectasis, pyelonephritis, osteomyelitis, TB, Hodgkin's disease.

A3   Investigations of a case like this require a comprehensive history, physical examination and laboratory investigations. This is a bad/difficult question, since causes include chronic disease as well as nutritional deficiency or chronic blood loss, and therefore it can lead anywhere. Investigation primarily addresses the identification of the nature of the anaemia so, for example, microcytic or macrocytic anaemia should be identified on a full blood count. In someone this age it is unlikely that a haemoglobinopathy would suddenly become apparent. Use this question as a basis for discussion in a tutorial with your teachers.

A4   Management depends on severity. The mainstay of treatment is inhaled salbutamol. In severe cases salbutamol should be given by nebulizer and steroids administered. Failure to respond may indicate the need for nebulized anticholinergics. In those not already using theophyllines, aminophylline may be given if the condition does not improve. Occasionally ventilation may be required.

A5 This is a difficult question requiring more common sense than hard fact, since the actual reason is unclear. Air polllution is often quoted but is not necessarily true and data are conflicting.

A6 Anticoagulation is of particular benefit if there is an increased risk of thromboembolic events, e.g. previous embolism, hypertension, left ventricular dysfunction, mitral valve disease. Probably not required in young patients if there is lone atrial fibrillation.

B1 Light chain fragments of immunoglobulins found in the urine.

B2 **Definition**: The permanent functional death of the centres in the brainstem that control the breathing, pupillary and other vital reflexes. Two independent medical practitioners are required to certify such a state.

C1

	Creatinine kinase	AST	LDH
Start to rise (hours)	4–8	6–8	12–24
Peak (hours)	12–24	24–48	48–72
Duration (days)	3–5	4–6	7–12

C2 *Vascular* – Haemorrhage/ischaemia;
Infective – Abscess;
Neoplastic – Primary, secondary, paraneoplastic;
Demyelination – Multiple sclerosis;
Toxins – Alcohol, anticonvulsants;
Hereditary – Freidreich's ataxia.

C3 *Cardiovascular* – Ischaemic heart disease, peripheral and cerebrovascular disease;

Respiratory – COAD/emphysema, bronchial neoplasm;

Gastrointestinal – Peptic ulceration, oral, oesophageal and gastric carcinoma.

C4 Autosomal recessive (1 in 2500 live births).

D1 Patients may use the adjective 'mild' to indicate that their condition is controlled by diet or oral hypoglycaemics alone.

D2 Be able to explain the principles: give 1 l of normal saline over 1 hour (watch in the elderly). Start intravenous insulin and give potassium. Monitor fluid balance, urea and electrolytes and blood sugar carefully. Identify precipitating cause, e.g. infection.

D3 Anorexia, yellow vision, nausea and vomiting, gynaecomastia, rhythm disturbances. Side effects are more likely if hypokalaemia or renal failure are present.

D4 Endoscopy is the method of choice. Biopsies are sometimes indicated to determine if *H. pylori* positive.

D5 *Helicobacter pylori* appears to play an important role but to say that the condition is an infective disorder is misleading. If *H. pylori* positive then antibiotic eradication is indicated.

E1 Conventionally, all four limbs. Chest leads are placed as follows:

V1 fourth intercostal space just to the right of the sternum

V2 fourth intercostal space just to the left of the sternum

V3 midway between V2 and V4

V4 fifth intercostal space in the midclavicular line

V5 left anterior axillary line at the same horizontal level as V4

V6 left midaxillary line at the same horizontal level as V4.

E2 Sinus tachycardia, 'S1 Q3 T3', right axis deviation, right bundle branch block.

E3 A syndrome arising from a congenital cardiac abnormality which initially has a left-to-right shunt, causes pulmonary hypertension and subsequent reversal of the shunt with consequent cyanosis.

E4 Erythrocyte sedimentation rate. Raised in a number of disease processes so therefore not of diagnostic benefit, but is useful in assessing disease activity.

F1 A type III hypersensitivity reaction to inhaled antigen (*Micropolyspora faeni, Aspergillus fumigatus, Thermoactinomyces vulgaris*) present in mouldy hay. It is one of the causes of extrinsic allergic alveolitis.

F2 Loss of the nailbed angle; excessive curvature of the nail in all directions; fluctuation of the nailbed.

F3 1. Immunosuppressed patients:
   cytotoxic drugs
   immunosuppressive drugs
   aplastic anaemia
   AIDS
2. Diabetics
3. Patients on broad-spectrum antibiotics.

G1 Antalgic gait (e.g. osteoarthritis)
Spastic paraparesis (e.g. cerebral palsy)
Spastic hemiparesis (cerebrovascular accident)
Cerebellar (most often seen at closing time!)
Unilateral foot drop:
   common peroneal nerve palsy
   polio (Inspector Morse)
Parkinsonian.

G2 A reliable and reproducible assessment of a patient's conscious level which has prognostic value. It assesses three responses: best motor response, best verbal response and eye opening.

G3 **Definition**: – An abnormality of uric acid metabolism causing deposition of urate crystals in the joints.

Treatment: Acute attack, NSAIDs.

Prevention: Allopurinol, weight loss, reduce alcohol intake, withdraw thiazides/salicylate if possible.

G4 *Congenital* – Klinefelter's (XXY).

Acquired: Normal puberty, chronic liver disease, malignancy (especially testicular, adrenal).

Drugs: digoxin, cimetidine, oestrogens, spironolactone.

H1 *Oesophageal:* Varices, erosive oesophagitis, Mallory–Weiss tear.

Gastric: Gastric ulcer, gastric cancer, erosive gastritis, gastric varices.

Duodenal: Ulceration, duodenitis.

H2 Bony swellings seen at the distal interphalangeal joints in osteoarthritis.

H3 Sweating, nausea and vomiting, tachycardia, altered behaviour, seizures, coma.

I1 Falling pulse, rising blood pressure, drowsiness, IIIrd/VIth nerve palsy, fixed dilated pupils, Cheyne–Stokes respiration, coma.

I2 Recurrent abdominal pain (usually in the iliac fossae) with diarrhoea and/or constipation but no demonstrable organic pathology. It is a diagnosis of exclusion and is more common in women. It may be associated with non-ulcer dyspepsia.

J1 Seizures which originate in the motor cortex, with jerking movements often arising first in the fingers or at the angle of the mouth and subsequent spread to the limbs on the opposite side to the seizure focus.

J2 Small non-tender erythematous macules seen in the hands in approximately 5% of cases of infective endocarditis.

J3 **Definition**: A raised serum bilirubin level, i.e. when the serum bilirubin exceeds 40 µmol/l. May be classified as prehepatic, intrahepatic or post-hepatic. An alternative classification is of elevated conjugated or unconjugated bilirubin.

J4 The venous pulse shows two positive pulsations for each cardiac cycle, compared to a single arterial pulsation. The venous pulse is more easily seen than felt and the arterial is more easily felt than seen.

K1 Polycystic kidneys may be detected through familial screening. Symptoms include loin or abdominal discomfort and haematuria. There may be hypertension or complications thereof, and there may also be uraemic symptoms.

K2 A feature of some dermatological conditions where skin lesions erupt in a linear fashion at sites of trauma, e.g. surgical scars, scratching.

L1 Small areas of cerebral infarction which are common in patients with hypertension and may be asymptomatic. Pure motor and sensory strokes are often the result of lacunar infarction.

L2 Suspect if hyponatraemia, lymphopenia, dry cough, confusion, diarrhoea and a prodromal viral-like illness.

L3 First described after an outbreak affected a Veterans' reunion in Philadelphia.

L4 Simvastatin (4S Study) and pravastatin (WOSCOPS Study) have respectively been shown to reduce mortality and incidence of myocardial infarction in patients with ischaemic heart disease and asymptomatic hypercholesterolaemia.

L5   Emphasis should be placed on treating those with risk factors for cardiovascular disease.

M1   *Causes of folic acid deficiency:* dietary, malabsorption, pregnancy.

   Causes of B_{12} deficiency: pernicious anaemia, gastrectomy, ileal disease.

   Other causes: alcoholism, liver disease, myxoedema.

M2   Reduce mortality by reducing incidence. Patient education to avoid exposure, wearing sunscreen and protective clothing are all important.

M3   *Symptoms:* malaise, fever, headache, photophobia and vomiting.

   Causes:

   Bacterial: *N. meningitidis, H. influenzae, Strep. pneumoniae, M. tuberculosis.*

   Viral: Echovirus, poliovirus, coxsackie virus, mumps, fungal, *Cryptococcus neoformans.*

M4   *Acute attack:* Paracetamol, NSAIDs, metoclopramide, ergotamine, sumatriptan.

   Prophylactic: Propranolol, diltiazem, pizotifen.

M5   The three diagnostic criteria are: paraproteinaemia, Bence-Jones proteinuria, lytic bone lesions.

N1   *Features:* heavy proteinuria, oedema and hypoalbuminaemia.

   Causes: Glomerulonephritis 80%, connective tissue disease (especially SLE), diabetes, amyloid, myeloma, drugs.

N2   Gastrointestinal irritation, fluid retention, exacerbation of asthma, nephrotoxicity, hepatotoxicity.

O1   An infection caused by an organism not usually responsible for causing illness but which may do so in the presence of impaired immunity in the host.

O2   Patients who suffer from old age, premature menopause, immobilization, steroid therapy, thyrotoxicosis, alcoholism, long-term heparin therapy.

P1   Aplastic anaemia, acute leukaemia, systemic lupus erythematosus, hypersplenism, marrow infiltration, pernicious anaemia.

P2   Paracetamol is converted to a toxic metabolite which causes hepatic cell necrosis and sometimes acute renal failure. Treatment is with *N*-acetyl cysteine. The best prognostic indicator is the prothrombin time.

P3   Principles of management include assessment of conscious state. If there is a gag reflex and the paracetamol has been taken within 4 hours then gastric lavage may be performed. Monitor vital signs and check paracetamol levels. Administer *N* acetyl cysteine. Intravenous dextrose should be given to prevent hypoglycaemia. Hepatocellular failure may require transplantation.

P4   *Transudate:* Cardiac failure, nephrotic syndrome, hepatic failure.
Exudate:
Infective causes: pneumonia, TB, subphrenic abscess. Malignancy. Pulmonary infarction.

P5   Iron-deficiency anaemia in association with an oesophageal web and, on occasions, a post cricoid carcinoma.

P6   Sit patient up, give 100% oxygen, diamorphine, intravenous frusemide and intravenous nitrate.

P7 Infection, lymphoma, leukaemia, connective tissue diseases, sarcoid, renal carcinoma.

Q1 A prolonged QT interval arises when ventricular repolarization is delayed, predisposing the patient to life-threatening ventricular arrhythmias.

Causes:

Congenital: Romano–Ward syndrome, Jervell–Lange–Nielsen (deafness).

Acquired: Electrolyte disturbance–low K, Mg, Ca; antiarrhythmics–Class 1a and 3; antipsychotics.

R1 **Definition**: A phenomenon caused by spasm of the arteries supplying the digits, characterized by pallor followed by cyanosis and reactive hyperaemia. It is associated with connective tissue diseases, beta-blockers and in individuals who work with vibrating tools.

R2 A condition most common in young men characterized by a triad of seronegative arthritis, non-specific urethritis and conjunctivitis.

R3 Briefly, rheumatoid arthritis is symmetrical and predominantly affects the small joints of the hand (metacarpophalangeal and proximal interphalangeal). Osteoarthritis usually affects the larger weight-bearing joints and the distal interphalangeal joints of the hand.

S1 A multisystem granulomatous disorder. Chest X-ray appearances include bilateral hilar lymphadenopathy and generalized pulmonary infiltration, which can progress to a honeycomb fibrosis pattern.

S2 The ideal screening test will have a low false negative and false positive rate. The disease which is being screened should be common and be prevented or more successfully treated by earlier detection.

S3 Shock can be defined as a failure of tissue perfusion resulting in cellular hypoxia. Causes: Hypovolaemic (e.g. haemorrhage, burns); cardiogenic (e.g. extensive infarction, cardiac rupture); sepsis; anaphylaxis.

S4 Immunosuppression, hypertension, hyperglycaemia, buffalo hump, poor wound healing, fluid retention, peptic ulceration, osteoporosis, cataract, psychosis.

S5 Main side effects are haemorrhage and allergic reactions. Contraindicated if recent (<14 days) trauma or surgery, stroke (<6 months), gastrointestinal bleeding or previous administration.

T1 Weight loss despite good appetite, sweating, tremor, dislike of heat, palpitations and diarrhoea.

T2 Increase organ donation by public awareness campaigns and carrying of donor cards. A controversial area is the issue of 'opting out' rather than the present opt-in system.

T3 Sharp, shooting 'electric-shock'-like pains precipitated by washing, shaving, combing hair, eating or cold weather. Treatment is with carbamazepine, phenytoin, amitriptyline or by ablation of the ganglion.

T4 TB may affect any organ. Clinical problems are seen in lung, kidneys, heart, GI tract, bone, skin, eyes, adrenals and the central nervous system.

T5 TB is more common in areas of poverty and overcrowding, among alcoholics and in immunosuppressed individuals.

U1 Perforation, perianal abscess, acute 'toxic' dilatation; extraintestinal involvement, colonic carcinoma.

U2 Poor prognosis is indicated by: >6 stools per day, fever, tachycardia, ESR >30, Hb <10 g/dl; albumin <30 g/l.

U3 *Cardiovascular:* Myocardial and valvular function, Doppler arterial studies.

Gastrointestinal: Gallbladder, liver, kidney, spleen and pancreas.

Genitourinary: Obstetrics, pelvic pathology, testicular masses.

Endocrine: thyroid.

V1 Zidovudine (AZT) inhibits HIV reverse transcriptase, so impairing viral replication and progression of the disease.

V2 *Vitamin A* – Night blindness, corneal dryness and ulceration.

Vitamin C – Weakness, muscle pain, spontaneous bruising/haemorrhage, scurvy.

Vitamin D – Impaired growth and rickets (children), osteomalacia (adults).

Vitamin E – Anaemia, haemolysis and muscle disorders.

Vitamin K – Clotting disorders.

Niacin – Pellagra (diarrhoea, dermatitis, dementia).

Riboflavin – Dermatitis.

Thiamine – Wet and dry beriberi.

W1 An encephalopathy associated with alcohol abuse, characterized by brainstem signs and irreversible amnesia.

W2 It is a rare inborn error of copper metabolism causing hepatic problems (cirrhosis), parkinsonian-type features and, if untreated, dementia.

X1 Duchenne muscular dystrophy, colour blindness, haemophilia A+B.

X2 Small pneumothorax; cervical rib; secondary deposits; hiatus hernia behind heart; subdiaphragmatic air; rib fractures; mastectomy.

Z1 It is a syndrome caused by a gastrin-secreting pancreatic tumour and characterized by peptic ulceration.

SURGERY

HISTORY AND EXAMINATION IN SURGERY

The standard method of history taking applies in surgery as in the other disciplines. The variety of conditions that present to surgeons is considerable, but general principles still apply. It is important to appreciate that underlying medical conditions may be an important determinant of the surgical treatment undertaken. Where relevant, such issues will be raised within the discussion of cases.

Abdominal masses commonly appear in surgical examinations, and in this section examination of the liver, spleen and kidneys will be considered in detail. The patient with ascites, with or without signs of chronic liver disease, is also a favourite with examiners, and so general examination is important.

There is no doubt, however, that at some time you will be required to demonstrate your skills in clinical examination of the abdomen. This may be done in almost any patient, even one attending for treatment of a ganglion if the examination organizer is having a bad time! Consequently this will now therefore be covered in some depth.

GENERAL EXAMINATION

Look for signs of anaemia (pallor, poorly injected conjunctivae etc. and jaundice (pay particular attention to the sclerae). Consider the other systemic signs of chronic liver disease, for example gynaecomastia, testicular atrophy, loss of body hair and spider naevi. Pay particular attention to the hands and look for clubbing, nail changes, palmar erythema and Dupuytren's contracture. The examiners may intervene and ask you to confine your examination to the abdomen itself, but at least you will have demonstrated logic in your thinking.

ABDOMINAL EXAMINATION

As for any system this should proceed in an orderly manner, i.e. inspection, palpation, percussion and auscultation.

Definitions

Abdominal masses commonly appear in surgical examinations, and these include:

Abdominal mass – any abnormal mass palpable on abdominal palpation.

Hepatomegaly – palpable enlargement of the liver.

Splenomegaly – palpable enlargement of the spleen.

Hepatosplenomegaly – enlargement of both liver and spleen.

Ascites – free fluid within the peritoneal cavity

Inspection

Look for any previous scars and describe them fully.

Ask the patient to cough. This has two functions: in the presence of a previous scar coughing may demonstrate an incisional hernia, and in any patient, their reaction to a cough tells you whether there is any peritonism, although this is unlikely in the exam.

Watch to see if the abdomen is moving with respiration. Are there any obvious masses? If so, does the mass move with respiration? An enlarged liver can usually be seen to do so.

Is there any abdominal distension? Remember that fullness in the flanks suggests ascites.

Are there any dilated veins on the abdominal wall? Veins radiating out from the umbilicus (caput medusae) are suggestive of portal hypertension, whereas dilated superior and inferior epigastric vessels may be indicative of inferior vena caval obstruction.

Palpation

You will immediately create a good impression with the examiners, irrespective of what findings you elicit, if you do the following:

1. Position the patient correctly.
2. Position yourself correctly.
3. Ask the patient if he or she has pain at any site before laying a hand on him or her.
4. Watch the patient's face throughout to witness their reaction.
5. Proceed in an orderly manner.

The patient should be placed supine, with only one pillow supporting the head. The entire abdomen should be exposed, including the groin, although it is customary to keep the genitalia covered. You must stand on the patient's right and position yourself such that your elbow is at the level of the patient, with the effect that your forearm and hand approach the patient's abdomen horizontally. If there is no chair present you will have to kneel on the floor to achieve this position. Begin with light palpation and proceed round all four abdominal quadrants in an orderly manner, watching the patient's face throughout. If he or she has indicated that one particular area is tender leave that quadrant until last. During this part of the examination you are largely gaining the patient's confidence, but you should note any guarding, tenderness or obvious masses.

All four quadrants are then palpated deeply, again with a flat hand but this time exerting more pressure. Sometimes it helps to place one hand over the other for this purpose. Both hands may be used to assess the size of any palpable structure. As before, ensure that you pay attention to the patient's reaction, particularly their facial expression, as this is often the best sign of local discomfort.

Remember that it is normal to be able to feel certain viscera, particularly in thin patients. Such structures include the sigmoid colon, the caecum, the aorta and the lower pole of the right kidney (compare with the left kidney which is impalpable unless diseased).

Deep palpation is followed by the examination of specific organs or for certain conditions as follows:

The liver
The anterior edge of the normal liver is occasionally palpable below the right costal margin. As the organ enlarges it extends down towards the right iliac fossa, hence when you are asked to palpate a patient's liver you should start here. The organ moves downwards with inspiration and use is made of this excursion during examination.

Palpation is carried out using the flat of the right hand placed across the right side of the abdomen. The upper edge of the hand is pressed deeply into the abdomen during expiration and maintained in that position while the patient inspires. A descending liver edge will be felt against the edge of the examining hand as the patient takes a deep breath in. If you are unable to feel the liver initially, then gradually work upwards towards the costal margin, each time moving the hand during expiration so that it is positioned deeply again before the patient inspires.

Record the size of the palpable liver in terms of centimetres or finger breadths below the costal margin in the midclavicular line. Note the character of its surface, its consistency and the presence or absence of tenderness.

Percussion can be used to confirm the position of the lower liver edge and is the only clinical method of determining the upper limit of the liver. Always percuss from resonant to dull in the midclavicular line, i.e. from below upwards in the abdomen and from above downwards in the chest. The upper border of the liver normally lies between the 4th and 5th intercostal spaces, but may be pushed downwards by conditions such as chronic obstructive airways disease.

The spleen

The normal spleen is impalpable. The organ has to be enlarged by a factor of two to three before it emerges from behind the left costal margin and extends downwards in the direction of the right iliac fossa.

Like the liver, the spleen moves downwards on inspiration and the same hand movements are used to palpate it, starting from the right iliac fossa and working towards the left costal margin. An 'equivocal' spleen may be made more obvious by rotating the patient on to their right side. The organ is characterized by its notched anterior border.

The kidneys

The left kidney is normally not palpable unless diseased, but occasionally the lower pole of the right kidney can be felt, especially in thin females. The kidneys are best felt between two hands, one placed in the loin pressing anteriorly and one on the abdomen pressing posteriorly. A palpable kidney may also be felt to descend on inspiration.

You should remember how to determine whether a left upper quadrant mass is kidney or spleen, as follows:

1. You can get your hand above the kidney, but not above a spleen.
2. A band of resonance is evident on percussion over the kidney but not over the spleen. Resonance is caused by gas in the colon.
3. The spleen has a notched anterior border.

Ascites

The presence of free fluid within the peritoneal cavity can be determined by either a demonstration of shifting dullness or a fluid thrill, and you should be familiar with both techniques.

Shifting dullness relies on percussion and, as always, you should percuss from resonant to dull, i.e. from the midline towards the flank. In general terms it is advisable to percuss the left side of the abdomen since the presence of an enlarged liver on the right side can mask the gas–fluid interface.

The hand in contact with the abdominal wall should be parallel to the midline and the point at which the percussion note changes from resonant to dull marked with a pen. The patient is then asked to roll on to their opposite side (i.e. normally the right side) following which you should wait a few moments to allow time for the intraperitoneal fluid to redistribute itself. Percussion is then repeated and if free fluid is present, the line of demarcation between resonant and dull will have moved.

To perform the test for a fluid thrill you need an assistant's hand, the ulnar border of which is placed lightly on the abdominal wall in the midline. The palmar surface of one of your hands is lightly laid on the lateral aspect of the abdomen while you 'flick' the abdominal wall on the opposite side with a finger of your other hand. If sufficient free fluid is present, the impulse generated by the sudden sharp contact of your finger is transmitted to the palpating hand as a fluid thrill. You may occasionally be asked what the purpose of the assistant's help is. You should know this, but it is, of course, to prevent transmitted pulsation over the abdominal surface.

The aorta

The aorta is normally palpable in the upper abdomen of thin subjects and there may be visible pulsation. An overlying mass may make aortic pulsation appear more prominent, and you should be aware of how to distinguish this from a palpable aorta or visible aneurysm. The key to this is that the pulsation of the aorta (or of an aortic aneurysm) is expansile (i.e. the pulse 'pushes' your two hands apart), whereas transmitted aortic pulsation is not expansile. To estimate the diameter of the aorta or an aneurysm, bring the radial borders of both hands together until you clearly feel the expansile pulsation, then subtract 1–2 cm from the distance between them to allow for the thickness of the patient's abdominal wall fat. Remember that the aorta bifurcates at approximately the level of the umbilicus, with the effect that the aorta can only be felt in the upper abdomen.

Auscultation
In the examination of the abdomen, a stethoscope will be most frequently employed for listening to bowel sounds. All you really need to be able to do is to tell if they are normal, absent (e.g. paralytic ileus or generalized peritonitis) or increased (intestinal obstruction). In the late stages of obstruction, when the bowel loops are distended, fluid-filled and atonic, there may be tinkling sounds caused by the movement of fluid from one distended loop to another. Remember that normal bowel sounds may be increased by a meal or by fasting.

Bruits caused by turbulent flow in a diseased aorta may be heard in the epigastrium. Be careful, however, that you are not simply hearing transmitted sound from a cardiac murmur. Disease in the iliac vessels may produce bruits along a line from the umbilicus to the midinguinal point.

The presence of a succussion splash in a fasted patient is diagnostic of pyloric stenosis. It is caused by excess fluid in a dilated stomach moving from side to side when you shake the patient. When present it can usually be heard without a stethoscope. A similar noise can be often elicited in a normal patient within a short time (1–2 hours) of a large meal or consumption of a large quantity of fluid.

THE CASES

ALTERED BOWEL HABIT (surgical aspects) ★★★★★

DEFINITION

A change in any aspect of defecation (frequency, stool consistency etc.) compared to what is regarded by the patient as 'normal'.

Causes:

- Colorectal cancer ★★★★★
- Diverticular disease ★★★★★
- Inflammatory bowel disease ★★★★★
- Infection ★
- Irritable bowel syndrome ★★★

HISTORY

You must establish what is regarded as the patient's 'normal' bowel habit, remembering that there is considerable individual variation in frequency of defecation. What is the time period over which the change has taken place? Has there been any possible precipitating cause (dietary change, travel abroad, new medication etc.)? Are there any associated symptoms (rectal bleeding, excess mucus, abdominal pain, tenesmus, weight loss etc.)? Is there a personal or family history of gastrointestinal tract disease?

EXAMINATION

General

Is there any evidence of recent weight loss or clinical signs of anaemia etc?

Abdominal

Is there any evident tenderness or abnormal palpable masses?

Rectal

Do not perform a rectal examination but you must say that you would like to do so. Specifically, you would be looking for any palpable abnormality or evidence of blood or mucus on the examining finger.

FACTFILE

1. Rigid sigmoidoscopy and double-contrast barium enema are the mainstay of diagnosis in the majority of cases.
2. The indications for flexible sigmoidoscopy and colonoscopy include confirmation of pathology suspected on barium enema (by biopsy), assessment of colitis (by direct visualization and biopsy), and the removal of polyps. Colonoscopy may also be selected in preference to barium enema as the first-line investigation in young patients to minimize pelvic irradiation, particularly in females.

DISCUSSION POINTS

1. In middle-aged and elderly patients the diagnosis is colorectal cancer until proven otherwise, and almost all instances merit further investigation.
2. In the young patient non-malignant causes are more common, but the possibility of carcinoma should not be discounted, particularly if there is a family history of the disease. You may be asked about familial bowel disorders.
3. You may be asked about the common symptomatology of bowel disease. Be clear what is meant by tenesmus, i.e. the constant sensation of the need to defecate and a feeling of incomplete evacuation.
4. Be familiar with the clinicopathological staging of colorectal carcinoma (Dukes') and its influence on prognosis.

5. You may be asked about the histopathological (and clinical) features that distinguish ulcerative colitis from Crohn's disease.
6. You may be asked how you would confirm the diagnosis of irritable bowel syndrome. It is important to emphasize that such a diagnosis can only confidently be made after the exclusion of significant organic disease.

HERNIAE ★★★★★

Patients with hernias are relatively easy to recruit for the examination. As a general rule they know what the problem is and what operation will be performed. It would be very rare to be presented with a patient with an acute complication of a hernia, but you should be aware of these.

DEFINITION

An external hernia is a protrusion of part of a viscus from the peritoneal cavity through a defect in the abdominal wall into an abnormal position.

Types of herniae

The following types of external herniae commonly appear in examinations:

- Inguinal ★★★★★
- Femoral ★★★
- Paraumbilical ★★★★
- Incisional ★★★★
- Epigastric ★★★

Rarer forms of external herniae which you are unlikely to encounter are:

- Obturator ★
- Spigelian ★

- Lumbar ★
- Sciatic ★
- Perineal ★
- Gluteal ★

TYPICAL PATIENTS

The most frequently encountered patients in undergraduate examinations are:

- Males (any age) with inguinal herniae ★★★★★
- Females (usually middle aged to elderly) with femoral herniae ★★★
- Patients of either sex (usually obese) with paraumbilical herniae ★★★★
- Patients of either sex with incisional herniae ★★★★

HISTORY

You should aim to identify symptoms related to the presence of a hernia, such as local discomfort, colicky pain (suggestive of intermittent intestinal obstruction) or the complaint simply of a 'lump coming out'. If the hernia is easily reduced then the lump may disappear overnight.

Risk factors should be identified: a history of chronic obstructive airways disease is important, since not only may a chronic cough may be the causative factor but its presence may influence management. Similarly, chronic constipation, prostatism, previous childbirth or previous surgery may be highlighted in the aetiology.

EXAMINATION

Groin herniae ★★★★★

This is the most common type of hernia to appear in examinations and the majority will be inguinal. The following questions need to be answered during the course of examination:

1. Is there a hernia present?
2. If so, is it reducible? (in examinations most will be)
3. Is the hernia inguinal or femoral?
4. If inguinal, is it direct or indirect?

Begin the examination with the patient lying supine. There may be an obvious bulge present, particularly if the hernia is irreducible. If not, ask the patient to cough and look for the typical bulge of a reducible hernia as the intra-abdominal pressure suddenly increases. If you still cannot see anything convincing, ask the patient to stand and repeat the above manoeuvres. The diagnosis is confirmed by feeling a cough impulse. To do this, place the fingers of the examining hand gently over the site of the hernia and ask the patient to cough.

Do remember that an irreducible hernia may not show any cough impulse.

To determine whether the hernia is inguinal or femoral you must examine to find out if the cough impulse is palpable above (inguinal) or below (femoral) the inguinal ligament, which runs from the anterior superior iliac spine to the pubic tubercle.

Correctly speaking, an inguinal hernia will emerge through the superficial inguinal ring, above and medial to the tubercle, whereas a femoral hernia will protrude through the femoral ring, which lies below and lateral to the tubercle. The tubercle itself, however, can be difficult to palpate in obese patients, although in the male you can usually feel the spermatic cord running over it.

The classic examination question should now be anticipated, i.e. is the hernia direct or indirect? Ironically, the answer to this makes little if any difference to clinical practice.

Chiefly you want to find out if finger pressure over the deep inguinal ring controls the hernia (indirect) or whether the hernia emerges medial to this point (direct). To do this you must first reduce the hernial sac. One finger is then placed over the deep inguinal ring (1 cm above the midpoint of the inguinal ligament), the other hand is laid gently over the medial part of the inguinal canal and the patient is asked to cough.

An alternative technique in the male is to invaginate the upper part of the scrotum through the superficial inguinal ring. When the patient coughs a direct hernia should be felt as an impulse against the posterior surface of the finger, whereas an indirect hernia, coming down the inguinal canal, will be felt against the tip. This technique can be useful for detecting small herniae but it is uncomfortable and best avoided except when necessary. Try the first technique and mention the alternative when the examiners ask if there is any other method that will distinguish between direct and indirect herniae.

It is important to examine patients with suspected herniae both supine and standing. Failure to do so may cause you to miss a hernia and will be criticized.

FACTFILE

1. The differential diagnosis of a groin hernia includes inguinal lymphadenopathy, sapheno varix, undescended or ectopic testis, hydrocoele of the cord, lipoma of the cord and femoral artery aneurysm.
2. Patients may present as an emergency. The usual cause will be that the hernia has become irreducible and/or obstructed and/or strangulated.

DISCUSSION POINTS

1. Treatment. The only effective form of treatment is surgical repair: trusses are only applicable to elderly patients who are unfit for operation. You may be asked to discuss this and how you would assess the patient.

2. It is only at operation that the nature of an inguinal hernia can be determined with certainty. Clinical examination is notoriously unreliable, and in any case operative confirmation of a clinically diagnosed direct hernia does not exclude there being an indirect sac present.

3. Be certain of the difference between an obstructed hernia (mechanical obstruction of the gastrointestinal tract) and a strangulated hernia (interruption of the blood supply).

4. Hernia surgery has undergone change, with a trend towards day case surgery, and alternative surgical techniques, such as laparoscopic repair, are becoming more popular.

Paraumbilical hernia ★★★★

True umbilical herniae occur only in infancy. The typical patient with an acquired paraumbilical hernia is obese and middle aged. Women are affected more often than men. The defect usually starts in the linea alba immediately above the umbilicus, and as the sac enlarges the umbilicus becomes distorted. Small herniae contain extraperitoneal fat but large sacs may contain small bowel or transverse colon. Large herniae are rarely reducible and are at risk of obstruction and strangulation. Operative repair is therefore advised, and this normally entails removal of the entire umbilicus.

Incisional hernia ★★★★

Think of this as a possible diagnosis whenever you are asked to examine an abdomen on which there is a visible surgical scar. The hernia may not be obvious with the patient lying flat, but will usually become apparent whenever you ask the patient to cough or to raise their shoulders off the bed.

You will probably be asked about predisposing factors to incisional herniae. These include poor surgical technique, wound infection, obesity, chronic cough etc., and factors which impair wound healing, (such as steroids, uraemia, advanced malignancy, hypoproteinaemia.

Epigastric hernia ★★★

This occurs in the midline through a small defect in the linea alba. It is most common in young fit males and normally comprises extraperitoneal fat, although occasionally a small peritoneal sac may be present. It is almost always irreducible and is usually easier to feel than to see.

JAUNDICE (surgical aspects) ★★★★★

DEFINITION

Yellow staining of the body tissue secondary to excess circulating bilirubin. It is classified as pre-hepatic (haemolytic), hepatic or post-hepatic (obstructive).

In a surgical ward or examination the most likely type of jaundice you will see is post-hepatic or obstructive. It is essential, however, that you are aware of how to determine the probable type of jaundice on clinical examination and history, and what investigations to arrange.

HISTORY

You must take a standard history of the presenting complaint and all other symptoms. Do not forget to ask about the colour of the urine. Remember that urine which is dark immediately it has been passed suggests the passage of conjugated bilirubin in obstructive jaundice.

Are the stools pale (reflects the absence of bile pigments in obstructive jaundice)?

Is the skin itchy (occurs in obstructive jaundice owing to the deposition of excess circulating bile salts)?

Is the patient known to have gallstones?

Is there a history of liver disease (e.g. viral hepatitis, primary biliary cirrhosis etc.)?

Is there a history of any haemolytic condition (e.g. spherocytosis, thalassaemia etc. Ethnic background is important)?

A past history of biliary tract surgery may not be mentioned by the patient.

A history of other significant disease is important. Some cases of hepatomegaly and jaundice result from metastases.

Ask (subtly) about alcohol consumption, but remember this may not be accurate. The drug history is important and a significant negative finding illustrating that you are aware of the hepatotoxicity of some agents and that others cause haemolysis or cholestasis.

EXAMINATION

1. Establish that the patient is jaundiced, remembering that the earliest signs are in the sclerae.
2. Are there any excoriations, suggesting itch?
3. Look for evidence of chronic liver disease.
4. Examine the abdomen, paying particular attention to the presence of ascites, hepatomegaly, a palpable gallbladder and any abnormal masses.

You will be asked about relevant investigations. You should have performed urine testing if a specimen is available.

FACTFILE

1. *Urine testing* Using standard multitest strips, this is easily performed in the ward. The presence of bilirubin indicates obstructive jaundice (or intrahepatic cholestasis), since only water-soluble conjugated bilirubin can pass through the glomerulus. Urobilinogen will be absent in total biliary obstruction, as this comes from the gut following bacterial action on bile products. Excess urobilinogen will, however, be present in haemolytic jaundice.

2. *Liver function tests* The bilirubin level will confirm jaundice and give an indication as to its severity. A disproportionately raised alkaline phosphatase is suggestive of biliary tract obstruction, whereas high levels of the transaminases (AST and ALT) are indicative of hepatocellular damage.

3. *Coagulation screen* Coagulation will be normal in prehepatic jaundice. The prothrombin time will be often be prolonged in obstructive jaundice but correctable with parenteral vitamin K. In severe hepatocellular disease both the PT and APPT will be prolonged and the former will not be corrected by vitamin K.

4. *Viral screen* This should be considered essential in all jaundiced patients.

5. *Imaging techniques* Ultrasound is the initial imaging modality in jaundice and can image the liver parenchyma, the intrahepatic and extrahepatic biliary trees, the gallbladder and pancreas. Computed tomography (CT) scanning or endoscopic retrograde cholangiopancreatography (ERCP) may be required in certain circumstances.

6. *Remember Courvoisier's law:* 'If in the presence of obstructive jaundice the gallbladder is palpable, then the jaundice is unlikely to be due to stones'. This rule relies on the premise that in gallstone disease the gallbladder wall is thickened and fibrotic and therefore unable to distend in the face of an obstructed biliary tree. A normal gallbladder, however, can become considerably distended when the distal obstruction is caused by a carcinoma in the head of the pancreas. The rule is, of course, not absolute, as clearly gallbladder disease and carcinoma can coexist.

DISCUSSION POINTS

You will almost certainly be asked about causes of obstructive jaundice and you should present them in their order of frequency. In the following list the first two conditions are responsible for the majority of cases.

- Gallstones
- Carcinoma of the head of the pancreas
- Nodes in the porta hepatis
- Bile duct tumours (cholangiocarcinoma)
- Benign bile duct strictures
- Sclerosing cholangitis.

RECTAL BLEEDING ★★★★★

DEFINITION

The passage of blood per rectum.

CAUSES

- Colorectal cancer ★★★★★
- Haemorrhoids ★★★★★
- Benign polyps ★★★
- Diverticular disease ★★★★
- Inflammatory bowel disease ★★★★★
- Anal fissure ★★★
- Ischaemic colitis ★★

HISTORY

Determine the nature of the bleeding, e.g. is it bright red, altered blood, clots, on toilet paper, in the pan or mixed with the stool? Bright red blood suggests an anal source, whereas altered blood and the passage of clots indicates a more proximal cause. Does bleeding only occur with defecation or does it necessitate the wearing of an incontinence pad? What is the timescale of the bleeding? Are there any associated symptoms, e.g. altered bowel habit, weight loss, tenesmus, abdominal pain etc?

DISCUSSION POINTS

1. Haemorrhoids are the most common cause of rectal bleeding, but must not be assumed to be the source of blood loss without consideration of more sinister pathology, particularly in the middle-aged and elderly age groups. Discussion may centre around investigation, and if your patient has haemorrhoids you must not agree with the examiners if they say that 'surely no further investigations need be done'.

2. Melaena (offensive black tarry stools) usually indicates an upper gastrointestinal tract source of blood loss but can occur with caecal lesions. Once again the methods of diagnosis and differential diagnosis will be discussed.

3. Remember that gastrointestinal bleeding can be sufficient to result in anaemia without being clinically obvious. Right-sided colonic pathology (caecal carcinoma, angiodysplasia) is a more common source of this type of blood loss than comparable conditions in the left colon. Such patients will have positive faecal occult blood tests. The role of faecal occult blood testing could arise in discussion.

SKIN LESIONS ★★★★★

Any abnormality arising from the skin or its adnexae may be found in the finals, usually as a short case.

Clearly, cutaneous abnormalities are too numerous to list in detail and only the common abnormalities likely to appear in examinations will be discussed here. It is important to remember that in the majority of cases the diagnosis can be made on the basis of clinical examination without the need to resort to biopsy.

EXAMINATION

Examination of a cutaneous lesion is no different from examination of an abnormality anywhere else in the body. Palpation is preceded by inspection, during which you should describe the appearance of the lesion, state whether it is solitary or multiple, and mention whether there is any other apparent abnormality. Palpation allows you to determine the size of the lesion, its consistency, whether it is well defined or diffuse, the presence or absence of tenderness, fixity to the skin or deeper structures etc.

COMMON ABNORMALITIES

Sebaceous cyst ★★★★★

Although not strictly correct, the term sebaceous cyst is usually applied to all cysts arising from pilosebaceous follicles. They are retention cysts which are caused by blockage of the duct of a sebaceous gland and are particularly common on the scalp, neck, face and scrotum. The cyst is filled with white/yellow 'cottage cheese' like material which is frequently foul-smelling. A central punctum will always be present, although it can sometimes be difficult to identify. The lesion is 'fixed' to the skin but mobile on the underlying structures. The vast majority can be excised under local anaesthetic. Occasionally sebaceous cysts become infected and either discharge spontaneously or require incision and drainage. Subsequent elective excision is required, as otherwise the recurrence risk is high.

Lipoma ★★★★★

Lipomas occur anywhere where there is fat, and are particularly common in the subcutaneous tissue of the trunk and limbs. Because fat is semiliquid at body temperature they present as soft fluctuant lesions and are usually well defined, although occasionally they can be diffuse. If unsightly or interfering with clothing they can be excised, usually under local anaesthetic. If large or extending deeply into intermuscular planes, a general anaesthetic may be necessary.

Dermoid cyst ★★★

Congenital dermoid cysts occur at sites of embryonic cleavage lines. These are seen most commonly in the midline of the neck, the angles of the orbit, on the abdomen or in the scalp. They present as unilocular cystic structures not attached to the skin. Congenital dermoids are lined with squamous epithelium and contain hair follicles, sweat glands and sebaceous glands.

Implantation dermoids are thought to arise from the implantation of epidermal cells beneath the skin by a penetrating injury. They occur most commonly on the hands and fingers and present as a subcutaneous cystic swelling. A scar may be visible to signify previous injury. The cyst is filled by whitish material and although lined by stratified squamous epithelium, skin appendages are always absent.

Ganglion ★★★★★

Ganglia present as subcutaneous cystic swellings and are seen most frequently on the dorsum of the wrist and less commonly around the ankle and dorsum of the foot. The cyst has a fibrous wall and contains a glairy viscous fluid. Usually they are asymptomatic, but occasionally they press on adjacent nerves and cause local discomfort and symptoms in the distribution of the nerve. The origin of ganglia is debatable. They are usually assumed to be due to herniation of synovial membrane from an adjacent joint or tendon sheath, but they may simply be degenerative lesions. Treatment is by excision under tourniquet control.

Neurofibroma ★★★

Neurofibromas are benign tumours arising from the neurilemma sheath. They can arise along the course of any peripheral nerve. They usually present in adult life as painless soft masses and are in many instances asymptomatic, although pressure may produce pain along the distribution of the nerve from which the lesion arises. Neurofibromas can be solitary, but the condition of multiple neurofibromatosis (Von Recklinghausen's disease) is inherited as an autosomal dominant characteristic and frequently accompanied by multiple café-au-lait spots on the skin. The latter condition may be associated with skeletal, endocrine or renal abnormalities.

Seborrhoeic keratosis ★★

Seborrhoeic keratoses are common benign skin lesions affecting the middle-aged and elderly. They are most common on areas of skin exposed to sunlight, such as the face, forearms and hands. They are frequently numerous and range considerably in size, from a few millimetres up to 2–3 cm. The appearances are also variable, from small yellowish spots to large warty plaques. On sebaceous gland areas they tend to be smooth, dome-shaped swellings with a central umbilication containing a keratin plug. Skin tags are probably a form of seborrhoeic keratosis affecting the neck and trunk, predominantly of middle-aged women.

Keratoacanthoma ★★

A benign tumour that originates from pilosebaceous follicles, keratoacanthomas occurs most frequently on the exposed skin of middle-aged and elderly men. It starts as a skin-coloured or reddish papule which rapidly enlarges over a 4–6-week period to form a smooth nodule 1–2 cm in diameter. Usually there is a central keratin-filled umbilication and some associated telangiectasia. Left alone, the lesion will regress spontaneously over a variable period (3–9 months) to leave an irregular, puckered scar.

Papilloma ★★★

Papillomas are benign epidermal tumours which can be pedunculated or sessile and are occasionally pigmented. A variant is the common wart, which is thought to be viral induced.

Basal cell carcinoma ★★★

This is the most common malignant skin tumour, but although it is locally destructive it rarely metastasizes. It is most common in fair-skinned individuals who have experienced long-term exposure to sunlight. Patients are therefore usually middle-aged or elderly and the majority of lesions occur on the face. Basal cell carcinomas usually begin as small translucent papules but progress to central ulceration with a raised, rolled edge. Treatment is either surgical (excision with or without skin grafting) or radiotherapy.

Squamous carcinoma ★★

Like basal cell carcinoma this tumour most commonly occurs on the exposed skin of fair individuals, but is more aggressive and can metastasize to regional lymph nodes and further afield. Squamous carcinoma may also develop in irradiated skin and at sites of chronic irritation, e.g. long-standing fistulae, sinuses and varicose ulcers (Marjolin's ulcer). The appearances may vary from an indurated ulcer to a fleshy fungating mass. Treatment may involve combinations of wide local excision, dissection of regional lymph nodes and radiotherapy.

Benign naevi ★★★

Benign naevi are rather variously described in textbooks. The common mole or intradermal naevus has no malignant

SURGERY

potential. Melanoma may, however, occasionally develop in a junctional or compound naevus.

Malignant melanoma ★★★

Melanoma is most common in fair-skinned individuals living in tropical climates, but its incidence has been steadily increasing in the UK. It is more common in females, particularly affecting the legs. Melanomas of the trunk, however, are more frequently seen in men. Macroscopically there are two common forms, superficial spreading or nodular. Superficial spreading melanoma is the variety where a long-standing pigmented lesion changes, for example in size, degree of pigmentation or symptoms (itching, bleeding etc.). Nodular melanoma does not arise from a pre-existing lesion but presents simply as a skin nodule. This latter type has a greater tendency for early invasion of the dermis. Remember also that melanoma can develop in the nailbed (subungual melanoma). The primary treatment is surgical and involves wide local excision with or without skin grafting. Amputation of the affected digit is indicated for subungual melanoma. The value of block dissection of regional lymph nodes remains controversial. The prognosis of malignant melanoma is related to the histological depth of invasion from the basal layer of the epidermis and the thickness of the primary lesion. Spread is predominantly by local skin permeation and lymphatic invasion. Haematogenous dissemination does occur but is usually a relatively late phenomenon.

STOMAS ★★★★★

You may be presented with a patient with a stoma, and this could be as either a long or a short case. In the former the history before the operation will obviously be important. In a short case you may only be asked to comment on the site and nature of the stoma, but do mention any other scars you see.

DEFINITIONS

A stoma is an artificial opening of the gastrointestinal or urinary tract on to the surface of the body. All the common stomas are sited on the abdominal wall and may be defined as follows:

- Colostomy ★★★★★ an opening of the colon
- Ileostomy ★★★★★ an opening of the small bowel
- Ileal conduit ★★★ an isolated loop of small bowel into which the ureters are implanted
- Urostomy ★ direct opening of one or both ureters on to the abdominal wall

Colostomy ★★★★★

This can either be an end colostomy or a loop colostomy. With the former a single lumen will be apparent, whereas with a loop colostomy both an afferent and an efferent limb will be present, hence the alternative term double-barrelled colostomy. Remember that although any part of the colon can be brought up to the surface of the abdominal wall after surgical mobilization, it is always easier to use either the sigmoid or transverse colons since their mesenteries result in mobility.

Most loop colostomies are created from transverse colon and are usually sited in the upper right abdomen, half-way between the umbilicus and the costal margin through the rectus abdominis muscle. If recently created (within 10 days or so) a bridge will normally be still in place. This consists of a plastic rod which is placed behind the loop to hold it up to the skin surface. End colostomies are most frequently seen in the left lower abdomen, formed from either the sigmoid or the distal descending colon. Such stomas are created as part of abdominoperineal resection of the rectum or Hartmann's procedure. Their normal site is half-way between the umbilicus and the anterior superior iliac spine, again in the line of the rectus muscle. Remember, however, that although these are the 'normal' sites for colostomies, both loop and end stomas can be created at different sites on the abdominal wall, so always inspect a colostomy carefully. A colostomy may be created with the intention of its being temporary or permanent. Permanent colostomies are almost always end colostomies. Temporary colostomies are usually loops, but may be an end stoma. For example, although the colostomy constructed during Hartmann's procedure is an end stoma, the possibility of later reanastomosis to the rectal stump exists.

Ileostomy ★★★★★

An ileostomy is immediately distinguishable from a colostomy by the fact that the bowel is everted to form a spout, which protrudes from the abdominal wall by approximately 2–3 cm. The purpose of the spout is to ensure that the effluent passes cleanly into the stoma appliance, thus minimizing skin contact, since small bowel content is extremely irritant to the skin. The colour and consistency of the material in the stoma appliance will also give an indication as to what type of stoma you are dealing with. The usual site for an ileostomy is in the right lower quadrant, but the mobility of the small bowel means that an ileostomy can be brought out with ease on the left side of the abdomen should this be more suitable for the patient. Most ileostomies are end stomas which have been created after a procedure such as total colectomy for inflammatory bowel disease. However, a loop or split ileostomy may be formed as a temporary measure to protect a newly created ileal pouch and ileoanal or colorectal anastomosis. Loop and end ileostomies are not as easy to distinguish as their colostomy counterpart. The proximal lumen is everted to form a spout as in an end ileostomy, and this tends to obscure the distal lumen which lies flush with the skin.

Ileal conduit ★★★

An ileal conduit is similar in site and appearance to an ileostomy. However, urine rather than small bowel contents will be present in the bag. Usually the bag will have a drainage tap on it so that it can be emptied without having to remove the appliance.

Urostomy ★

Urostomies are more frequently used in children and are uncommon in adults. Their appearance may vary considerably. One ureter may be brought out in the flank with the other anastomosed to it retroperitoneally. Alternatively, both ureters may be brought out together in the midline of the abdomen, giving a double-barrelled appearance.

DISCUSSION POINTS

You may be asked about preoperative preparation of a patient who requires a stoma. It is important that stomas are appropriately sited and that skin creases are avoided to minimize the chances of leakage. Once the site is chosen it is marked with an indelible pen so that it can be clearly identified in the operating theatre. Factors to be considered when preparing the patient include age, occupation, type of clothing worn, lifestyle and hobbies (swimming etc.) and the presence of any physical disabilities which may inhibit self-care of the stoma (e.g. visual impairment, arthritis etc.). Psychological preparation of the patient and postoperative support are also essential. In most centres much of this work will be carried out by dedicated stoma care nurses.

UPPER ABDOMINAL PAIN ★★★★★

You are unlikely to see a patient presenting with acute pain, so the majority of conditions seen will be chronic.

DEFINITION

Abdominal pain above the level of the umbilicus.

COMMON CAUSES

- Gallbladder disease ★★★★★
- Gastro-oesophageal reflux ★★★★★
- Duodenal ulcer ★★★★
- Gastric ulcer (benign or malignant) ★★★
- Pancreatic disease ★★★

HISTORY AND EXAMINATION

As for pain in any other part of the body you must determine the exact site, radiation, severity, character, associated features, precipitating and relieving factors. In many instances, once you have done this you should have a good idea as to the likely cause of the patient's symptoms. It is important to remember that rarely are any patient's symptoms 'typical' of a condition, but the following may help to determine the underlying problem.

Gallbladder disease ★★★★★

Frequent complaints are of upper abdominal pain, predominantly epigastric and right upper quadrant, which can radiate around to the back, the interscapular area or the right shoulder tip. During attacks the patient is often restless and unable to find a comfortable position. Often they complain that their symptoms are precipitated by eating, and are accompanied by nausea and flatulence. Spontaneous resolution occurs after a variable period of time. These symptoms are frequently labelled as biliary 'colic', although they are more likely to reflect gallbladder distension rather than true colic. A separate clinical entity is acute cholecystitis, where there is mucosal inflammation and ulceration secondary to cystic duct obstruction. Local discomfort and tenderness is a feature of this condition, with systemic signs of toxaemia. On examination look for any evidence of jaundice. Check for tenderness or a palpable gallbladder in the right upper abdominal quadrant, often exacerbated by deep inspiration (Murphy's sign). Upper abdominal ultrasound is the first investigation of choice.

Gastro-oesophageal reflux ★★★★★

The typical patient will describe burning epigastric discomfort which radiates retrosternally. The symptoms will often be worsened by stooping or on lying flat. A foul bitter taste is also commonly described. There may be a history of mild haematemesis. Antacids (often bought over the counter rather than on prescription) may have been used to obtain relief of symptoms. Endoscopy is the investigation of choice.

Duodenal ulcer disease ★★★★

The most common complaint of patients with chronic duodenal ulcer disease is epigastric pain, which is precipitated by fasting and relieved by food or antacids. Not infrequently patients are woken from sleep by their symptoms. Sometimes the discomfort radiates through to the back, and certain foods such as spicy meals or alcohol may aggravate matters. There may be a history of intermittent vomiting or previous haematemesis. Weight loss is uncommon in uncomplicated duodenal ulcer disease, but symptoms of anaemia may develop from chronic upper gastrointestinal blood loss. On examination, look for clinical signs of anaemia and check the abdomen for any palpable abnormality and tenderness. Investigation is by upper gastrointestinal endoscopy.

Gastric ulcer ★★★

Patients with gastric lesions frequently complain of a gnawing discomfort and vague dyspepsia. These symptoms are often constant and not affected by food or antacid mixtures. Profound anorexia is a common complaint, particularly in patients with malignant disease, and consequently weight loss is a frequent feature. Intermittent vomiting and minor haematemeses are not uncommon. Proximal gastric cancers may result in dysphagia, whereas pyloric canal lesions can lead to gastric outlet obstruction. General examination should include a check for signs of anaemia, weight loss and lymphadenopathy in the supraclavicular regions. When considering the abdomen you may need to determine whether a succussion splash is present, or whether there is any evidence of ascites. Palpate the abdomen and note if there is an upper abdominal mass, tenderness or palpable hepatomegaly. Investigations include barium meal and endoscopy and biopsy.

Pancreatic disease

Acute pancreatitis ★

You will not see an acute case but may see a patient recovering from the acute episode.

DEFINITION

A condition characterised by autodigestion of the pancreas by its own escaped enzymes.

CAUSES

- Gallstones
- Alcohol
- Viral (e.g. mumps, Coxsackie)
- Trauma (including surgery)
- Drug-induced (steroids, thiazide diuretics)

- Hypercalcaemia
- Hypothermia
- Idiopathic

The first two causes are responsible for the vast majority of cases.

HISTORY

The patient will usually have presented as an acute surgical emergency following the sudden onset of severe constant upper abdominal pain which frequently radiates through to the back. Often patients find sitting with the knees drawn up to the chest the most comfortable position to adopt. Vomiting and retching are a common accompaniment. There may be a history of long-standing chronic alcohol excess or of 'binge' drinking. Alternatively, there may be a history of gallstone disease.

EXAMINATION

In an examination you will not be asked to examine a patient in the acute phase of pancreatitis but you may be taken to see someone who was admitted with the condition several days previously. On general examination, take note of the patient's general demeanour. Do they look comfortable or distressed? Is there any evidence of jaundice? Do they have a temperature? Is there any evidence of chronic liver disease? Extravasation of blood in haemorrhagic pancreatitis may cause discoloration around the umbilicus (Cullen's sign) or in the flanks (Grey Turner's sign). On abdominal palpation you would not be surprised to find some tenderness and guarding in the epigastrium, but note also whether there is any palpable mass. The abdomen may be generally distended if an ileus persists. The absence of bowel sounds will confirm this.

DISCUSSION POINTS

1. **Diagnosis** is based on measurement of the serum amylase. A level above 1000 IU/l is confirmatory.
2. **Assessment of severity** The amylase level gives no indication as to the severity of the disease. You should be aware of Imrie's (or Ranson's) criteria for assessment of the severity of the condition. Mild cases almost invariably settle with conservative management. On the other hand severe acute pancreatitis is a serious condition with appreciable morbidity and mortality rates.
3. **Investigations** All patients should undergo ultrasound examination of the pancreas and biliary tree to look for gallstone disease. In gallstone pancreatitis there is increasing evidence that early ERCP with sphincterotomy and clearance of the common bile duct can alter the course of the disease. Patients with severe acute pancreatitis will require a dynamic contrast-enhanced CT scan to look for evidence of pancreatic necrosis.
4. **Complications** These are almost always confined to the severe prognostic group and include infected pancreatic necrosis, pancreatic abscess and pseudocyst formation.
5. You may be asked about long-term sequelae such as malabsorption and diabetes.

VARICOSE VEINS ★★★★★

DEFINITION

Varicose veins are dilated, tortuous, lengthened superficial veins.

Patients used for examination purposes will usually have varicosities of the long saphenous venous system with readily demonstrable saphenofemoral incompetence. Short saphenous problems and recurrent varicose veins rarely appear in undergraduate exams.

HISTORY

Determine the symptoms that prompted referral. These include cosmetic appearance, aching or discomfort, typically towards the end of the day or after prolonged standing, ankle swelling and skin problems such as eczema or ulceration. A family history may be relevant, as will a past history of pregnancies or previous deep venous thrombosis.

EXAMINATION

Inspection

1. Are there any skin changes (eczema, ulceration, pigmentation, lipodermatosclerosis etc.)?
2. Which part of the superficial venous system is varicose (long or short saphenous)? If long saphenous, is there a visible varix over the saphenofemoral junction? Is there any evidence of a varix overlying one of the constant medial leg perforators, signifying perforator incompetence? This part of the examination must clearly be done with the patient standing.
3. Are there any scars suggestive of previous surgery?
4. Are there any immediately obvious predisposing factors (e.g. pregnancy)?

Special tests

1. Is there a palpable thrill (or bruit on auscultation) over the saphenofemoral junction when the patient coughs?
2. The tourniquet or Trendelenburg test is the definitive clinical test of varicosities. The affected limb is elevated and the varicosities emptied. A tourniquet is then placed around the thigh with the aim of preventing superficial venous filling from above. It is important at this stage to ensure that the tourniquet is sufficiently tight and that it is placed around the thigh as high as possible, so as to be close to the saphenofemoral junction. If the varicosities

are entirely due to saphenofemoral incompetence then a properly applied tourniquet will prevent any filling. Filling from below indicates perforator incompetence and you have then to work your way gradually down the leg repeating the test until the level of venous incompetence is demonstrated.

FACTFILE

1. Treatment options include support, as provided by a properly fitted elasticated stocking. Support is particularly useful in cases where other forms of treatment would be contraindicated e.g. in pregnancy and the unfit elderly patient.

2. Injection sclerotherapy is the technique most applicable to minor cosmetic varicosities below the knee or for residual varicosities following surgery. The technique involves injecting the sclerosant (usually either ethanolamine or sodium tetradecylsulphate (STD)) into the emptied varicosity and then maintaining compression on the leg for 2–3 weeks. Problems include skin ulceration if care is not taken to ensure that the injection is intravascular.

3. The aims of surgery are to correct deep to superficial venous incompetence and to remove unsightly varicosities. For saphenofemoral incompetence this involves groin exploration, ligation of all the tributaries of the upper long saphenous vein, and ligation and division of the long saphenous vein flush with the femoral vein. Perforator incompetence requires ligation and division of the relevant perforating veins. Other varicosities can be removed by stripping or by stab avulsions.

DISCUSSION POINTS

1. You may be asked about the special investigations of venous function. These include Doppler examination and, on occasion, venography.

2. You may be asked about specific risk factors for varicosities and invited to discuss how these might be alleviated.

LEG ULCERS ★★★★

These can be seen as long cases but are frequently seen as short cases.

DEFINITION

An area of skin breakdown on the lower limb.
Common types are:

- Venous (responsible for 70–80%) ★★★★★
- Ischaemic (arterial) ★★★★
- Traumatic ★★

Infrequent types are:

- Infective ★★★
- Neoplastic ★★★
- Neuropathic ★★★

EXAMINATION

Describe the ulcer with respect to its site on the limb, its size, the nature of the edge, appearance of the base (e.g. slough, granulation tissue etc.), and the presence or absence of surrounding erythema or cellulitis. Pay attention to the appearance of the entire limb. Does the patient have varicose veins? Are there any signs of chronic ischaemia (pallor, hair loss, nail changes, absent pulses etc.)? Is there evidence to suggest peripheral neuropathy? Are there signs of infection in the limb (cellulitis, lymphangitis)?

FACTFILE

Venous ulcers ★★★★★

1. These are most commonly found overlying or just above the medial malleolus. Often there will be other skin changes associated with superficial venous hypertension, such as eczema and induration and pigmentation of the skin (lipodermatosclerosis).
2. Venous ulcers can occur without a history of previous deep venous thrombosis and in the absence of gross superficial varicosities.
3. Treatment may involve surgery, where feasible, to correct the superficial venous hypertension, and dressings with compression bandages to promote ulcer healing. Resistant cases may require admission to hospital for enforced bed rest.
4. In long-standing cases, squamous carcinoma can develop at the edge of the ulcer (Marjolin's ulcer).

Arterial (ischaemic) ulcers ★★★★

1. These are most commonly seen on the lateral aspect of the leg, the dorsum of the foot, the toes or the heel.
2. Other signs of peripheral vascular disease will almost certainly be present.
3. There may be scars from previous arterial surgery.
4. Even in a short case look for corroborative evidence of aetiology and, if time allows, comment, for example, on tar staining of the fingers.

Traumatic ulcers ★★

1. These ulcers most frequently occur where there is little tissue between the skin and underlying bony prominences (e.g. over malleoli, anterior tibia and the posterior aspect of the heel).
2. Pretibial lacerations are common injuries in elderly patients who fall. This type of injury tends to raise a flap of skin with the base distally. Healing is slow owing to the limited blood supply to this area.

DISCUSSION POINTS

1. If a varicose ulcer is kept above heart level it will heal
   – a fact, but often not achievable in clinical practice!
   The management of these ulcers is difficult and you may
   be asked about what you have seen and how they have
   been treated.
2. 'Patient education may be one of the most important
   factors in prevention and treatment of varicose ulcers.'
   You may be asked to comment on this kind of statement.
   This can be difficult but does provoke discussion.

NECK LUMPS (excluding the thyroid) ★★★★

Neck lumps commonly appear as short cases in both undergraduate and postgraduate examinations and are frequently
a cause of great concern to candidates. Textbooks tend to give
rather daunting lists of differential diagnoses. This section is
intended to simplify the approach to the examination and
diagnosis of the more common types of lump to appear in
surgical finals.

DEFINITION

Neck lumps should be described in terms of their anatomical distribution and may be midline, in the anterior triangle
(i.e. anterior to the sternomastoid muscle) or in the posterior
triangle (i.e. posterior to the sternomastoid).

Lumps must be also described with respect to all the
criteria normally applied to any lesions e.g. size, shape,
character, mobility, tenderness etc. In the neck, lumps superficial to the investing cervical fascia are no different from
lumps elsewhere in the body, and comprise sebaceous cysts,
lipomas, neurofibromas etc. More specific lesions, many of
which are peculiar to the neck, lie deep to the cervical fascia
and it is these that are discussed here.

SURGERY

MIDLINE NECK SWELLINGS

Midline swellings are solitary lumps which arise from unpaired midline structures.

The two most common are thyroglossal cysts and midline dermoids.

Thyroglossal cyst ★★

This is the most common midline neck swelling and usually presents as a painless, rounded cystic lump which moves on swallowing or protruding the tongue. It can occur anywhere along the thyroglossal tract, i.e. from the foramen caecum to the thyroid isthmus, but is uncommon above the hyoid bone. The cyst is freely mobile and the majority transilluminate. Occasionally they become infected and present as a thyroglossal fistula.

Midline dermoids ★★

These usually present as painless solid or cystic masses anywhere between the suprasternal notch and the submental region. The feature which distinguishes them from a thyroglossal cyst is that they do not move with protrusion of the tongue or with swallowing.

SWELLINGS IN THE ANTERIOR TRIANGLE

These occur in the space bounded anteriorly by the midline and posteriorly by the sternomastoid muscle. Lesions to be considered here include:

Thyroid lumps ★★★★, which are covered elsewhere, and branchial cysts.

Branchial cysts ★★

The majority of branchial cysts present in the upper part of the anterior triangle in young adults. The presenting features are variable. Most patients are aware of a continuous swelling but occasionally it can be intermittent. Pain occurs in approximately 30% of cases.

The typical branchial cyst is soft and fluctuant to palpation and can be felt extending out from the anterior border of the sternomastoid. Transillumination can rarely be elicited owing to the depth of the cyst in the neck. Treatment is by surgical excision.

Pharyngeal pouch ★

This is a pulsion diverticulum which emerges through the dehiscence of Killian between the thyropharyngeus and the cricopharyngeus on the posterior aspect of the pharynx. Usually the swelling appears on the left side of the neck. Pharyngeal pouches may be asymptomatic or may present with dysphagia and regurgitation.

Salivary gland swellings ★★★

These can be caused by inflammation, tumour or duct obstruction.

Mumps is the most common inflammatory cause. The commonest salivary gland swelling due to tumour is the pleomorphic adenoma, which occurs most frequently in the parotid gland as an asymptomatic firm unilateral swelling.

Facial nerve paralysis and a history of pain are important observations and should alert you to the possibility of malignancy.

Truly malignant tumours of these glands more commonly affect the submandibular and minor salivary glands. Duct obstruction by stone is more likely in the submandibular glands than the parotid.

Lymph nodes ★★★★★

Cervical lymphadenopathy may result from inflammatory or neoplastic conditions. Remember to look for lymphadenopathy elsewhere. Consider the possibility of tuberculosis, particularly in high-risk groups.

Carotid body tumours ★

Never mention these unless you are prepared to explain that they are tumours of the chemoreceptor apparatus at the carotid bifurcation. They tend to be oval and non-tender. They have lateral mobility but cannot be moved upwards or downwards.

Cervical rib ★

These are palpable in the supraclavicular fossa and may be associated with neurological or vascular symptoms. There are other miscellaneous causes but these need not be among your differential diagnoses.

SWELLINGS IN THE POSTERIOR TRIANGLE ★★★★★

The commonest cause of swelling in the posterior triangle is lymphadenopathy.

FACTFILE

1. The most common cause of neck lumps is lymphadenopathy.
2. Inflammatory or reactive nodes are usually tender.
3. The exception to (2) above is tuberculosis, where the infection is chronic and tenderness is uncommon.
4. Cervical lymphadenopathy is very common in children.
5. Palpable lymph nodes in adults should be regarded as pathological until proven otherwise.
6. In adults the primary cause of neoplastic neck lymphadenopathy is usually in the head or neck, and ENT examination is mandatory.

SCROTAL LUMPS ★★★★

DEFINITIONS

Hydrocoele ★★★★ a collection of fluid within the tunica vaginalis

Epididymal cyst ★★★★ single or multilocular cyst lying within the epididymis

Varicocoele ★★★★ an abnormal dilatation of the pampiniform plexus

EXAMINATION

When presented with a scrotal swelling there are a number of questions you need to ask yourself as you proceed with the examination:

1. Can I get above the swelling? If not, then it is likely you are dealing with a large indirect inguinal hernia.
2. Is the mass solid or cystic? Solid masses include testicular tumours ★ and chronic epididymo-orchitis. ★★★ (Acute epididymo-orchitis is extremely tender and therefore unlikely to appear in an examination.) Cystic masses are likely to be either hydrocoeles or epididymal cysts.
3. Can the testis be felt separately from the mass, and if so what is the relationship of the testis to it? With an epididymal cyst a normal testis will be palpable anteriorly. In tense hydrocoeles it is often difficult to feel the testis, but when it is palpable it will be posterior to the swelling. The testis will feel normal in the presence of a varicocoele but will be irregular if the diagnosis is a testicular tumour.
4. Does the mass transilluminate? This is a characteristic feature of hydrocoeles but some large epididymal cysts also transilluminate. This technique may help to confirm the relationship of the testis to the mass.

5. Is the abnormality altered by posture? Varicocoeles become visible and much more easily palpable as a 'worm-like' collection on standing. Remember that varicocoeles are almost invariably left-sided.

FACTFILE

1. Hydrocoeles may either be primary ★★★★ (no obvious cause) or secondary ★ to an underlying testicular tumour or testicular/epididymal infection. The possibility of tumour should always be considered in the younger patient and the testis fully assessed clinically and by ultrasound. Tumour markers (alpha-fetoprotein (AFP) and human chorionic gonadotrophin (HCG)) should be measured in such patients.

2. Testicular tumours are rare below the age of 20 and above the age of 40. Between these two ages, however, they are one of the most common malignancies and usually present as a painless testicular mass with or without an associated hydrocoele. The majority fall into one of two categories:

   (a) Seminoma: A homogeneous tumour which occurs most commonly in the 30–40-year-old age group. It spreads via lymphatics accompanying the testicular vessels to para-aortic lymph nodes. Treatment comprises inguinal orchidectomy, radiotherapy to the para-aortic nodes (the tumour is radiosensitive) and, increasingly, chemotherapy with platinum-based regimens.

   (b) Teratoma: The peak incidence of this tumour is in the 20–30-year-old age group and it is derived from tissue from all three germ layers. Teratoma has a tendency for haematogenous dissemination, and not infrequently presents as symptomatic lung metastases. Treatment requires orchidectomy and chemotherapy (cis-platinum). It is less radiosensitive than seminoma.

THYROID PATIENTS ★★★★

Typically the patient will be attending for operation on or assessment of the thyroid. Usually they will have one of two problems, i.e. a solitary thyroid nodule or multinodular goitre.

HISTORY

You should try to determine whether there are any symptoms of under- or overactivity of the thyroid and, if so, their duration. A past history of thyroid problems is not uncommon and there may be a family history of autoimmune disorder.

Symptoms of laryngeal nerve involvement (chiefly hoarseness) are important, as are stridor and dysphagia, which suggest tracheal and oesophageal obstruction.

EXAMINATION

General

Look for evidence of thyroid overactivity (e.g. tremor, sweating, tachycardia, weight loss, nervousness) or underactivity (weight gain, puffy eyelids, pretibial myxoedema etc.). Pay particular attention to the eyes in cases of suspected hyperthyroidism (lid lag, exophthalmos etc.).

The neck

Inspect the neck from the front. Is there any obvious thyroid enlargement (goitre)? If so is it diffuse or is there asymmetry between the two thyroid lobes? If there is any doubt about the nature of a solitary lump ask the patient to swallow. Is there any evidence of cervical lymphadenopathy? Palpate the thyroid gland, standing behind the seated patient. Ensure that the patient's neck is slightly flexed. Carefully palpate both lobes of the gland and the isthmus and determine whether you are dealing with a solitary nodule or a multinodular gland. Flexing the neck and rotating the head towards the side being palpated will relax the sternomastoid muscle and facilitate palpation of the individual lobes As during inspection, ask the patient to swallow while you palpate the gland (there will usually be a glass of water sitting nearby). Finally, palpate the neck and supraclavicular fossae for evidence of lymphadenopathy.

FACTFILE

1. Papillary carcinoma is the most common thyroid tumour in young adults and carries a favourable prognosis, with 5-year survival figures in excess of 90%. It usually presents as a solitary thyroid lump, although it is occasionally diagnosed following excision of a lymph node mass. The traditional surgical approach is total thyroidectomy combined with removal of any involved lymph nodes. Radioiodine scanning is then done and any uptake taken to represent occult metastases. In such instances therapeutic radioiodine is then administered. As the tumour is TSH dependent, surgical treatment is followed by suppressive thyroxine therapy.

2. A thyroid scintiscan may help to determine whether a nodule is solitary or part of multinodular change. It also identifies whether a solitary nodule, either does or does not take up iodine i.e. the 'hot' or 'cold' nodule but this is of limited value in surgical practice. Radioiodine uptake studies are sometimes used to make a functional assessment of thyroid gland activity in cases of borderline hypo- or hyperthyroidism.

3. The indications for surgery in patients with a multinodular goitre are autoimmune thyroiditis (e.g. Hashimoto's disease), diagnostic concern, pressure symptoms (e.g. stridor or dysphagia) or cosmetic (large unsightly goitres). Otherwise these conditions are normally treated conservatively.

4. Ultrasound assessment of the thyroid allows identification of the size and shape of the gland as well as distinguishing between cystic and solid lesions.

DISCUSSION POINTS

1. You may be asked about the particular investigations you would undertake in thyroid disease.
2. Treatment options are important, and you should know the indications for a surgical or medical approach to the patient with thyroid disease.
3. The risks of thyroid surgery are often discussed.

   (a) *Nerve damage:* The recurrent laryngeal nerves are intimately related to the lateral aspects of the thyroid gland and therefore at risk during thyroid lobectomy. In experienced hands the incidence of nerve injury is, however, low (<1%). Unilateral recurrent laryngeal nerve damage causes weakness and hoarseness of the voice. Bilateral paralysis is potentially life-threatening, in that it may result in laryngeal stridor necessitating tracheostomy. The external laryngeal nerve may be damaged while mobilizing the superior thyroid poles. This nerve innervates the cricothyroid muscle, paralysis of which affects the tension of the vocal cords and hence the timbre of the voice. Less commonly, the internal laryngeal nerves may be traumatized. This leads to desensitization of the appropriate side of the larynx, which can cause problems with fluids or secretions spilling over.

   (b) *Hypoparathyroidism:* Transient asymptomatic hypocalcaemia is common after thyroid surgery. Total thyroidectomy represents the greatest risk in terms of permanent hypoparathyroidism, but in experienced hands with parathyroid gland identification and preservation, the incidence of this should be low.

   (c) *Bleeding:* This is probably the best-known complication of thyroid surgery. If bleeding occurs deep to the cervical fascia the expanding haematoma can obstruct the airway and cause progressive respiratory embarrassment. In such instances opening the wound in the ward and evacuating the haematoma may be life-saving, but such dramatics are rarely required.

4. You may be asked about the different histological types of thyroid carcinoma and should know the basics of this.

TOENAILS ★★★★

Problems related to toenails commonly appear as short cases.

DEFINITIONS

1. The ingrown toenail ★★★★★
   This is the most common abnormality. Pressure necrosis between the nail, the nailbed and the edge of the nail sulcus leads to ulceration, inflammation and infection. Predisposing factors include tight footwear and cutting the nail too short with a curve at the edges.

2. The overgrown nail ★★★★
   Proliferation of the nail leads to its becoming elongated, curved and thickened. The resulting appearance is often described as horn-like. The alternative name for this condition is onychogryphosis.

3. Nailbed abnormalities
   The three most common conditions under this heading are:

   (a) *Subungual haematoma* ★: here trauma, usually of a crushing nature results in a tense, painful haematoma underneath the nail. Such cases should not be seen in the examination.

   (b) *Subungual exostosis* ★★: in this condition there is a small overgrown spicule of bone on the dorsal surface of the distal phalanx which causes upward pressure on the nail and may lead to deformity.

(c) *Subungual melanoma* ★★: Malignant melanoma can occasionally arise in the nailbed. A pigmented lesion will be visible through the nail. This condition should be considered in cases of undiagnosed groin node lymphadenopathy.

FACTFILE

1. Either conservative or operative treatment might be used in cases of ingrown toenails, although the former is only applicable if there is no persistent pain or infection.

2. Outpatient surgical treatment for ingrown toenails is the norm. This is usually done under a local anaesthetic block (a ring block). *Avulsion of the nail* simply involves removing the nail, and is essential to allow drainage of pus when infection is present. The nail will regrow, but with proper care and attention many patients will experience no further trouble. Commonly, therefore, this is recommended as the primary procedure in young patients, particularly females.

   Nailbed ablation to prevent regrowth of the nail is indicated for recurrent ingrown toenails. The two techniques employed are either surgical excision of the part of the nailbed responsible for nail growth, or chemical ablation using phenol. With phenol ablation the entire nail can be removed and the bed ablated, or the ablation can be confined to one side of the nailbed if only one corner of the nail is involved (wedge excision).

3. Treatment of onychogryphosis: This is normally treated by avulsion of the entire nail followed by ablation of the nailbed, either surgically or using phenol.

4. Treatment of a subungual melanoma: Following histological confirmation, amputation of the digit is the usual course of action.

BREAST LUMPS ★★★

Breast lumps are very common and may therefore readily be encountered in the examination. Remember that you may also be presented with a patient admitted for cholecystectomy who fortuitously has a breast lump. If you have identified this and the clinicians were unaware of it, then you are at something of an advantage for the remainder of the examination.

HISTORY

Generally the patient will already know about the reason for this attendance and you should identify how aware she is of the potential problems. Find out how she noticed the lump, and whether there was any nipple discharge and whether this was bloodstained. The identification of specific genes associated with familial cancers makes a family history essential, as is the reproductive history in terms of parity and whether she breastfed her children. The use of hormones, either the oral contraceptive pill or hormone replacement therapy, should be documented.

Questioning should be directed at the likely problems faced by particular women. Thus a young woman of 30 or less is more likely to have a fibroadenoma (★★★★), whereas the older woman may have a palpable breast cancer (★★★).

EXAMINATION

Inspection

Ensure that the patient is undressed from the waist up and sitting comfortably on an examination couch or bed. Look for any asymmetry between the two breasts, making allowances for normal slight variations in size. Are there any obvious lumps present? Are there any skin changes, such as tethering (areas of dimpling), ulceration or oedema (responsible for the *peau d'orange* appearance in advanced breast cancer). Pay particular attention to the nipples. Are they at the same level and of the same appearance? If one or other is inverted, establish whether it is recent or of long standing. Bilateral slit-like nipple inversion commonly occurs in association with the benign condition duct ectasia, whereas recent unilateral nipple indrawing may signify an underlying carcinoma. Is there evidence of nipple or areolar eczema, which may indicate Paget's disease? Finally, is there any evidence of bruising or a small incision suggesting percutaneous needle biopsy? Then ask the patient to elevate her arms above her head. This may make skin tethering or lumps more obvious. In addition, as a breast fixed by tumour to the chest wall will be less mobile, this will accentuate any asymmetry. Any abnormality should be described with respect to its position in the breast. Imagine the breast as comprising four quadrants divided by vertical and horizontal lines through the nipple.

Palpation

This should be done with the patient lying supine and with the arms by the side. Make a point of asking the patient if she is quite comfortable. Try to gain her confidence: if you seem too nervous then she will also be tense, making examination more difficult.

Ensure that you examine the patient in an orderly sequence, e.g. normal breast, affected breast, normal axilla and then that of affected side, both supraclavicular fossae and both sides of the neck.

Palpate the breast quadrant by quadrant initially with the flat of the hand. Begin with the 'normal' breast so that you get an impression of what is normal for the patient before moving to the affected side. If a lump is felt then palpate it between forefinger and thumb and describe it with respect to its site, size, shape, consistency, definition of margins and tenderness. Deep fixation to the pectoralis major should also be assessed. To do this, ask the patient to place her hands on her hips and alternately press down and relax while you move the lesion at right-angles to the direction of the pectoralis fibres (i.e. from inferolateral to superomedial and vice versa). The right axilla is examined with the left hand and the left axilla with the right hand. The non-examining hand is used to support the weight of the patient's arm. Begin by gently palpating the medial wall of the axilla and then gradually advance the examining hand towards the apex. Both supraclavicular fossae and both sides of the neck are then palpated for any evidence of lymphadenopathy.

FACTFILE

1. Fine-needle aspiration of breast lumps can provide a rapid diagnosis which can be available in the outpatient clinic. The experience of both surgeon and pathologist is important for accuracy.

2. Treatment of early breast cancer comprises local treatment directed at the breast and axilla (surgery and radiotherapy) and adjuvant therapy (chemotherapy and hormonal treatment).

3. The choice between mastectomy and lumpectomy will be influenced by a number of factors, including the size of the lesion in relation to the size of the breast, the site of the lesion and patient and surgeon preference.

   Following lumpectomy, radiotherapy is directed at the breast to reduce the incidence of local recurrence. It is not required after mastectomy unless the tumour was large with skin and/or muscle involvement. Radiotherapy will be directed at the axilla if tumour-positive nodes are identified there during *sampling*. If axillary *clearance* has been undertaken the risk of lymphoedema is increased and further damage by radiotherapy is avoided.

---

4. Tamoxifen (a competitive oestrogen antagonist) is of proven benefit in postmenopausal women in terms of reducing the risk of recurrence, prolonging survival and reducing the risk of a second cancer developing in the opposite breast. It is therefore standard practice to prescribe tamoxifen to all postmenopausal women following surgery. The efficacy of tamoxifen in premenopausal women is currently being assessed. Tamoxifen may also be used as a primary treatment in elderly women who are unfit for surgery or who have inoperable disease.

DISCUSSION POINTS

1. The examiners will want to know that you are aware of the differential diagnosis of breast conditions. Be aware of these and do not immediately start with small print, for example Tietze's syndrome.
2. The role of clinical and radiological screening programmes might be raised. Remember that because of the tissue density in younger women mammography is chiefly of use only in older women.
3. When discussing breast lumps it is possible that examiners will move on to other topics, such as the side effects of chemotherapy or terminal care.
4. It is likely that increasing recognition of markers for the risk of breast cancer, such as BRCA1, will lead to a greater interest in studying those women with a family history.

DYSPHAGIA ★★★

DEFINITION

Difficulty in swallowing.

COMMON CAUSES

- Benign oesophageal stricture
- Oesophageal carcinoma
- Achalasia of the cardia

HISTORY

You must establish the following:

1. Where does the food stick?
2. What type of foods are causing difficulty, solids alone or solids and fluids? If solids alone, is it certain types of food? Patients will usually have difficulty initially with dry materials such as bread. With total dysphagia, patients will have difficulty swallowing saliva.
3. Is the dysphagia progressive, and over what period of time? Rapidly progressive symptoms are suggestive of malignant pathology, whereas long-standing difficulty only with dry bulky foods would be more in keeping with benign disease.
4. Are there any other symptoms, such as weight loss, pain, respiratory disease, voice changes?
5. Is there a past history of reflux oesophagitis, which predisposes to stricturing?
6. Has the patient been treated previously, for example by dilatation?

EXAMINATION

1. General. Is there evidence of weight loss? Is the patient clinically anaemic?
2. Is there any palpable lymphadenopathy in the root of the neck or supraclavicular fossae?
3. Are there any abnormalities on abdominal palpation, in particular an epigastric mass or hepatomegaly?

Investigations
- Barium swallow
- Upper GI endoscopy
- Chest X-ray

DISCUSSION POINTS

1. The investigation of dysphagia is basic and you will almost certainly be asked about the differential diagnosis.
2. Dysphagia may provoke discussion about Barrett's oesophagus.

EQUIPMENT ★★★

You may be presented with a number of different instruments for comment. Alternatively, you may be asked to comment on 'equipment in use'. Thus your patient may have a chest drain *in situ* or a central venous line. You should be aware of the indications for these techniques and the complications that may arise from their use.

Particularly popular instruments to quiz students on include (for indeterminate reasons) sigmoidoscopes, proctoscopes and urinary catheters. Equally popular, though marginally more aesthetic, is the Sengstaken or Minnesota tube. These are exam favourites. In most institutions it will be a four-lumen Minnesota tube you are given. They are usually red in colour, with the gastric and oesophageal balloons being yellow/brown. If you look closely at the opposite end from the balloons you will see that the lumina are labelled, i.e. gastric balloon, oesophageal balloon, oesophageal lumen, gastric lumen.

Also included here, but not conventionally considered as equipment, are items such as temperature charts. These are another examination favourite. They can be discussed in their own right or they can form part of the examination when looking at individual patients.

DEFINITION

TPR chart This stands for temperature, pulse and respiratory rate. Often, however, respiratory rate is not marked but blood pressure will be included on the chart. If the patient has a surgical procedure, sometimes you will see written along the top of the chart Th, 1, 2, 3 etc., signifying the theatre day and subsequent postoperative days.

Postoperative pyrexia ★★★

If the chart shows a postoperative pyrexia the following should be considered:

1. **Basal atelectasis** This is the most common cause of a significant temperature rise on the first postoperative day in elective surgical patients (clearly, septic patients who have undergone emergency surgery have other reasons for being pyrexial). It is one of the commonest postoperative complications, affecting over 50% of patients in general surgical practice. Basal atelectasis is defined as basal alveolar collapse, and arises through a combination of hypoventilation and increased viscous secretion, which tends to block the small airways. The clinical picture may vary from the mere presence of the pyrexia to significant respiratory distress. Treatment requires adequate analgesia to permit coughing and full

respiratory effort, physiotherapy, and oxygen if required. Antibiotics are *not* required in the first instance as the pyrexia is caused by an inflammatory reaction and not infection. Properly treated, the patient's temperature will return to normal after 24–48 hours. If inadequately treated, however, infection will supervene and a pneumonia develops.

2. **Chest infection** An established chest infection tends to result from untreated atelectasis and usually presents around the 3rd to 4th postoperative days. The early pyrexia fails to resolve but increases, often with an associated tachycardia. Treatment requires physiotherapy, antibiotics and oxygen therapy.

3. **Wound infection** Surgical procedures can be classified as clean (no contamination and no visceral opening, e.g. varicose veins, hernias, breast operations), potentially infected (opening of a viscus, e.g. GI tract surgery, cholecystectomy) or frankly contaminated (e.g. laparotomy in a patient with a GI tract perforation). In clean operations the organism will usually be staphylococcal, coming from the patient's skin or the skin or nose of theatre staff. In the potentially infected category the mechanism of infection is bloodborne. A transient bacteraemia occurs on entering the relevant viscus and it therefore follows that the causative organism is dependent on the type of surgery, e.g. coliforms for large bowel surgery. In either case, clinical evidence of infection is unlikely to occur until at least 5–7 days postoperatively. Apart from the pyrexia, symptoms may include wound tenderness, erythema, a purulent discharge or superficial wound dehiscence.

Wound infection is an almost inevitable complication in a patient with a frankly contaminated peritoneal cavity, for example following colonic perforation.

4. **Intra-abdominal infection** This may take the form of either a localized collection or generalized peritoneal contamination arising from breakdown of a gastrointestinal tract anastomosis. In the latter condition the patient will usually have a fairly constant fever and will exhibit other signs of sepsis. The typical pattern associated with a localized collection (abscess) is a spiking pyrexia. The peaks may reach 40°C, at which point rigors are common. Almost normal temperatures may be recorded between these episodes.

Remember that the most common sites for intraperitoneal collections are the subphrenic spaces, the subhepatic space and the pelvis. All these areas can be visualized by ultrasound, which is therefore the investigation of choice. Pelvic collections may, however, be palpable at rectal or vaginal examination. An elevated hemidiaphragm, perhaps with an air–fluid level beneath it or a sympathetic effusion above it, may signify a subphrenic collection, particularly if the patient complains of shoulder-tip pain.

5. **Deep venous thrombosis** This may be associated with a low-grade pyrexia and usually presents on around the 10th postoperative day. Other clinical signs of venous thrombosis will often be present.

6. **Urinary tract infection** This is common in all patients undergoing major surgery and tends to be associated with urethral catheterization. It may cause a pyrexia from approximately the 3rd postoperative day onwards. If the catheter is still *in situ* the patient will often be asymptomatic, but the urine will usually be cloudy and contain visible debris. If the catheter has been removed the patient usually experiences the typical symptoms of a urinary tract infection (frequency, dysuria etc.). Infection should be proven by urine culture, however, as often the simple irritant effect of catheterization will lead to similar symptoms.

7. **Thrombophlebitis** Staphylococcal infections are not uncommon around intravenous cannulae and, if not dealt with, can lead to local suppuration and a spreading superficial thrombophlebitis. Venous access sites should therefore always be inspected in a patient with a pyrexia.

ORTHOPAEDIC CASES ★★★

Since orthopaedics is taught as part of the undergraduate curriculum it is not unreasonable to expect that they will appear in the surgical finals, usually as short cases. The following is a brief summary of some of the more common conditions to expect.

PERIPHERAL NERVE INJURIES

Radial nerve injury ★★★

The most common injury is fracture of the humerus involving the spiral groove. The nerve damage results in wrist drop, owing to paralysis of the extensors of the wrist. Sensation is impaired over the radial half of the dorsum of the hand, although often the sensory impairment can be minimal owing to overlap from the median and ulnar territories.

Median nerve injury ★★★

The median nerve can be damaged by blunt trauma resulting in fractures around the elbow or wrist, or by lacerations to the forearm. The level at which the damage has occurred will to some extent affect the clinical presentation. With all median nerve injuries there will be sensory loss over the palmar aspect of the thumb, and the lateral two and a half fingers. Sensation will also be lost over the dorsum of the distal phalanges of these fingers. There will be weakness and wasting of the muscles of the thenar eminence and the patient will be unable to abduct the thumb from the hand. Opposition of the thumb to the fingers is therefore impeded and the function of the hand significantly impaired. With proximal median nerve injuries the pronators of the forearm and flexors of the wrist and fingers will be paralysed. The exceptions to this are the flexor carpi ulnaris and the medial half of the flexor digitorum superficialis, which receive their innervation from the ulnar nerve. The unopposed action of these muscles in such an injury tends to lead to ulnar deviation of the wrist.

Ulnar nerve injury ★★★

Like the median, the ulnar nerve can either be damaged by fractures around the elbow or by lacerations to the forearm or wrist. The paralysis associated with ulnar nerve damage is characteristic as it supplies all the intrinsic muscles of the hand, with the exception of the three muscles of the thenar eminence (abductor pollicis brevis, opponens pollicis and flexor pollicis brevis) and the lateral two lumbricals. The hand therefore takes on a 'claw' appearance owing to the unopposed action of the long flexor and extensor muscles of the fingers. If the injury is at elbow level, paralysis of the flexor carpi ulnaris tends to produce radial deviation of the wrist, and paralysis of the medial half of the flexor digitorum superficialis means that clawing of the fourth and fifth fingers tends to be less marked. In terms of sensory loss, the patient will be numb over the palmar aspects of the fifth and the medial half of the fourth fingers. On the dorsum the distribution of the sensory loss can be similar or may extend to the third finger.

Common peroneal nerve injury ★★★

The common peroneal or lateral popliteal nerve can be relatively easily damaged where it winds round the neck of the fibula, either by fracture of the bone or by pressure from a tight plaster cast. Paralysis of the ankle and foot dorsiflexors and the peroneal muscles leads to foot drop and inversion respectively. Sensory loss occurs over the anterior and lateral aspects of the lower leg and foot. Sensation is preserved on the medial side, as this area is innervated by the saphenous nerve.

CARPAL TUNNEL SYNDROME ★★★

This condition is most common in middle-aged and elderly women and in pregnancy, and is caused by compression of the median nerve where it passes beneath the flexor retinaculum. The symptoms are of tingling and numbness in the hand over the territory supplied by the median nerve (see median nerve injuries above) and weakness of the muscles of the thenar eminence. Often the patient will complain of clumsiness of the hand. The tingling and discomfort are often worst at night.

HALLUX VALGUS ★★★★

In this condition there is lateral deviation of the great toe at the metatarsophalangeal joint. In most instances the first metatarsal is deviated medially, with the effect that there is a large gap between the first two metatarsal heads (metatarsus primus varus). After a period of time a bursa forms over the protruding head of the first metatarsal (the bunion), which may become inflamed. A later event is the development of osteoarthritis at the metatarsophalangeal joint. Hallux valgus is seen most frequently in middle-aged and elderly women, in whom the wearing of tight pointed shoes in the past may be relevant. Mild cases require only attention to the bunion and advice on appropriate footwear. If the disability is significant, surgery is indicated.

EXAMINATION OF THE HIP ★★★★

The hip is one of the joints you are more likely to be asked to examine. Students are often unsure of how best to perform the examination (as are most general surgeons), and the following is intended as a simplified guide.

Inspection

The patient should be lying supine, exposed except for underwear. First determine the lie of the legs relative to the pelvis and, if possible, square the pelvis. Look for evidence of scars suggesting previous surgery, sinuses, skin changes or any obvious deformity. Note the soft tissue contours for evidence of muscle wasting.

Palpation

Feel the bony contours for any irregularity and watch the patient's face for evidence of local tenderness. Skin temperature may give an indication of underlying inflammation.

Measurement of leg lengths

Here you need to be able to demonstrate and compare the true length of each leg, and also assess whether there is any apparent or false discrepancy which arises from sideways tilting of the pelvis. All limb measurements must be performed with the patient's legs placed parallel and as square to the pelvis as possible.

True leg length is measured from the anterior superior iliac spine to the medial malleolus. A tape measure is fixed at each of these bony points and the two sides compared.

'False' leg length is measured from a fixed midline structure, for example the xiphisternum, to the medial malleolus, and again the two sides are compared.

Examination for fixed deformity

Fixed deformities are caused by contraction of muscle groups or of the joint capsule. This may occur in arthritic conditions, and the most common deformities are adduction, flexion and lateral rotation.

Fixed adduction will have already been noticed when trying to place the legs parallel and square to the pelvis. A fixed adduction deformity makes this impossible. If you imagine a horizontal line drawn between the two anterior superior iliac spines (transverse axis of the pelvis) in normal circumstances a limb can be placed at right-angles to it. This cannot be done with fixed adduction, and the affected limb will lie at an acute angle to your 'line'.

Fixed flexion is assessed by Thomas's test. If a patient has a fixed flexion deformity he will compensate for it by arching the spine to allow the affected limb to lie flat. The effect of the spinal arch can be cancelled by fully flexing the unaffected limb, thus highlighting the flexion deformity. To do the test, with the affected limb placed flat on the couch assess the degree of lumbar lordosis by using your hand to measure the gap between the patient's lumbar spine and the surface of the couch. If no gap exists there can be no flexion deformity and you do not need to proceed further. If there is a lordosis, however, the unaffected limb is flexed to its normal limit and then forced further to push the lumbar spine down on to the couch. As this is done the affected limb will be lifted from the couch and the angle of the deformity can be measured.

Fixed rotation The rotational position of the hip is judged by the orientation of the patella. This should normally point forwards with the hip lying at rest. In the presence of a fixed rotation deformity, the hip cannot be rotated to get the patella into this neutral position.

Range of movements

Flexion, abduction, adduction and rotation are separately assessed and one leg compared with the other. With flexion and abduction/adduction it is important to discriminate true hip movement from pelvic movements. Therefore, when assessing flexion, one hand moves the limb while the other is placed on the iliac crest to detect any pelvic rotation.

Similarly, when testing abduction and adduction, the non-examining hand and forearm are used to bridge the two anterior superior iliac spines to determine whether any pelvic tilting is occurring.

Power

The power of all the relevant muscle groups should be tested by assessing their strength when contracting against resistance. As always, the two sides should be compared.

Postural instability

The Trendelenburg test is an assessment of the ability of the hip abductors (gluteus medius and minimus) to stabilize the pelvis on the femur. Under normal circumstances, when humans stand on one leg the hip abductors on that side tilt the pelvis to lift the non-weight bearing leg clear of the ground. If the function of the abductors is impaired they are unable to tilt the pelvis against body weight and the pelvis will tilt downwards on the side of the lifted leg. When performing this test always assess the 'normal' side before moving to the affected limb, but remember that the limb under test is the weight-bearing side, not the lifted leg.

Gait

Gait should be fully assessed by observing the patient walking.

EXAMINATION OF THE KNEE ★★★★

This should proceed in a logical manner similar to that described for examination of the hip.

Inspection

As described for the hip.

Palpation

Again, looking for the same features as described above.

Measurement of thigh girth

The important factor is the bulk of the quadriceps muscle. Measurements must be taken at exactly the same level on each side, in order to make an accurate comparison (measure up from the patella to ensure this).

Assessment of an effusion

The fluctuation test is the most accurate test of an effusion. One hand is placed over the front of the knee joint, with the thumb and index finger extending just beyond the opposite patellar margins. The other hand is used to exert pressure immediately above the patella on the suprapatellar pouch. If fluid is present fluctuation will be felt between the two hands. The alternative technique is the patellar tap, where you try and 'knock' the patella off the surface of the femur, but this is less reliable.

Assessment of movement

The only movements at the knee joint are flexion and extension, the range of which can vary considerably from patient to patient. In assessing movement, take note of any discomfort or crepitus.

Assessment of power

As for all other joints this is measured against resistance, one leg being compared with the other.

Assessment of stability

The stability of the medial and lateral ligaments is tested with the knee in a position just short of full extension With the knee fully extended a taut posterior joint capsule may mask ligamentous laxity. With the muscles relaxed, one hand takes the ankle while the other hand is placed behind the knee. The proximal hand is moved around each side of the joint in turn to stabilise the knee as the distal hand moves the leg to stress the joint. The cruciate ligaments are tested with the knee flexed to 90° and the foot fixed on the couch (usually by the examiner partially sitting on it). Grip the upper tibia with both hands (which come together posteriorly) and alternately pull and push the upper end of the tibia to determine how much gliding movement occurs between the tibia and the femur. Remember that the anterior cruciate prevents anterior movement of the tibia on the femur, whereas the posterior ligament has the opposite effect (the draw sign).

Rotation tests

McMurray's test is used to test for tears of the menisci and is dependent on the torn part getting caught between the femur and tibia. When the knee is straightened a loud click accompanied by pain indicates the meniscal tag being freed. The test involves flexing the knee, rotating the tibia on the femur (laterally then medially), and extending the knee while the tibial rotation is maintained.

Gait

As for the hip joint, analysis of the gait pattern is an important part of assessment of the knee.

TRIGGER FINGER AND TRIGGER THUMB ★★★

A common condition of unknown cause which leads to thickening of the fibrous flexor sheath at the base of the finger or thumb. The result is narrowing of the mouth of the sheath and swelling of the tendons immediately proximal to it. The swollen part of the tendon can only be forced into the mouth of the sheath when the digit is straightened from the flexed position. The patient usually complains of discomfort at the base of the affected digit and locking of the digit in full flexion, which usually has to be overcome by extending the digit passively with the other hand. Often there will be a palpable nodule at the base of the affected digit, which reflects the swollen part of the tendon.

DUPUYTREN'S CONTRACTURE ★★★★

This condition is caused by thickening and contraction of the palmar aponeurosis. The effect of this is to pull the fingers into flexion at the metacarpophalangeal and the proximal interphalangeal joints. Usually the fourth and fifth fingers are the most obviously affected, and the thickened aponeurosis is palpable.

The condition is of unknown causation, but it is more common in men and exhibits a degree of hereditary pre-disposition. The incidence is increased in association with liver disease, alcoholism and anticonvulsant drugs. Effective treatment requires surgery in which the palmar aponeurosis is excised.

PERIOPERATIVE CARE ★★★

DEFINITION

The preoperative preparation and postoperative care of the surgical patient. You may be asked in an examination how you as a pre-registration House Officer would manage a patient at ward level.

PREOPERATIVE PREPARATION

The following should be considered under this heading:

ECG

In most circumstances anaesthetists will want to see a pre-operative ECG in all patients over the age of 40 before general anaesthesia, and in younger patients if clinically indicated. Any history of significant cardiac disease may require a more detailed cardiovascular assessment.

Chest X-ray

The policy regarding preoperative chest X-rays will largely be determined by the anaesthetic department. In general, however, routinely performed chest X-rays are of little value and they need only be performed if clinically indicated. Such indications would include a history of cardiorespiratory disease, chest signs on clinical examination, and patients with malignant disease to look for possible metastatic spread.

Blood cross-matching

You will not necessarily need to be familiar with the different policies for blood cross-matching, but you should think logically if asked. To say that you would merely group and retain serum for a patient undergoing repeat hip replacement would be foolish.

Bowel preparation

Most surgeons prefer the colon to be mechanically cleansed before elective large bowel surgery. This can be done in a number of ways, including colonic washouts via a rectal catheter, gut irrigation by means of solutions taken orally, and stimulant laxatives such as Picolax. Care must be taken with the latter, as any significant degree of mechanical obstruction may result in perforation of the bowel. In obstructed cases it is usually safer to maintain the patient on an elemental diet and restrict mechanical preparation to rectal washouts.

Antibiotic prophylaxis

Antibiotic prophylaxis is not normally required for 'clean' procedures but should be considered for the potentially infective cases. It is normal practice to cover procedures such as biliary tract and gastrointestinal tract surgery, with the aim of reducing the risk of wound infection. The aim is to have a high circulating level of the appropriate antibiotic at the time surgery is carried out. This is usually best achieved by administering a dose intravenously at the time of induction of anaesthesia. Many surgeons will follow this up with two postoperative doses (e.g. at 6 and 12 hours) for large bowel cases. Clearly the antibiotic used must cover the likely infective organism, and in most instances broad-spectrum cover will be employed. Cephalosporins are commonly used, with the addition of metronidazole to cover anaerobes for large bowel surgery.

Prophylaxis against venous thrombosis

All patients undergoing major surgery are at risk of deep venous thrombosis. These risks are increased by a number of factors, including previous thrombosis, obesity, smoking, malignant disease, pelvic surgery and certain drugs, e.g. the oral contraceptive pill. Unless contraindicated, therefore, all patients should be considered for prophylaxis against venous thrombosis in an attempt to avoid the potentially fatal complication of pulmonary thromboembolism. Prophylaxis against venous thrombosis can be considered under the headings of general measures and specific measures.

General measures
- Preoperative weight reduction
- Early postoperative mobilization
- Avoidance of pressure on the legs at the time of surgery
- Graduated compression stockings
- Encouragement to stop smoking
- Delaying elective surgery for at least 6 weeks after stopping the oral contraceptive pill.

Specific measures
- Subcutaneous heparin
- Intraoperative pneumatic calf compression using specially designed 'boots'.

- Intermittent electrical calf muscle stimulation during surgery.

Miscellaneous

Valvular heart disease Patients with valvular heart disease require antibiotic prophylaxis to minimize the risk of endocarditis. In addition to any procedure-related antibiotics, it is normal practice to administer a combination such as gentamicin and amoxycillin at induction of anaesthesia.

Anticoagulant therapy Patients may be on regular warfarin therapy for a number of reasons, including prosthetic heart valves, atrial fibrillation, previous arterial embolism or venous thrombosis. Clearly the warfarin effect must be reversed to permit safe surgery, but at the same time a degree of anticoagulation may be essential, particularly in the patient with prosthetic cardiac valves. In such instances heparin is used, as this has a much shorter half-life than warfarin and is therefore more controllable.

POSTOPERATIVE CARE

This may include the following:

Haematology and biochemistry

Patients on intravenous infusions should have their biochemistry checked daily. It is normal practice to check the haemoglobin level the day following major surgery, although the figure on the second postoperative day will often be a more reliable guide to whether blood transfusion is required.

Analgesia

Adequate analgesia is important, not only on humanitarian grounds but also because it will permit coughing, deep breathing, cooperation with the physiotherapist and early mobilization, all of which help to reduce the risks of pulmonary complications and deep venous thrombosis.

Traditionally, analgesia following major surgery has involved regular intramuscular opiate injections, but recent years have witnessed a trend towards the use of epidural anaesthesia and patient-controlled analgesia (PCA). The last technique employs a pump which is programmed to deliver a specific dose of opiate intravenously whenever the patient presses a button. For safety reasons the device is set to deliver a maximum amount of drug per unit time, irrespective of the patient's demands.

Oxygenation
The majority of patients suffer a degree of respiratory depression postoperatively and supplementary oxygen may be required. This is of particular importance in patients with myocardial disease. It should also be considered for patients undergoing colonic resection, as the delivery of well oxygenated blood is important for anastomotic healing.

Fluid balance
Many a junior doctor has been kept out of bed worrying about what fluids to prescribe postoperatively. It is important to emphasize that in the majority of cases a central venous line is not necessary, and that the key to successful fluid balance lies in clinical assessment.

PERIPHERAL VASCULAR DISEASE ★★★

This section will address the issues of peripheral vascular disease as they affect the lower limbs. This is because you are more likely to be presented with a case of lower limb ischaemia with intermittent claudication than upper limb ischaemia. You should be aware of how the upper limbs may be affected, however, though the same general principles apply.

ACUTE ISCHAEMIA ★

Acute ischaemia is a surgical emergency and you will therefore not encounter such patients in examinations. You may, however, still be asked to take a history from and examine a patient who presented with this condition.

HISTORY

The patient complains of the sudden onset of severe pain, usually with numbness and loss of function of the affected limb. A history of trauma will be self-evident, either of an injury to the limb or iatrogenic problem (e.g. surgery or arteriography). You need to ask about previous symptoms of arterial insufficiency and about possible sources of embolism (valvular heart disease, arrythmias etc.). A patient with a past history of intermittent claudication who spontaneously develops acute ischaemia with no obvious source of embolism is likely to have suffered an acute occlusion. On the other hand, in someone with atrial fibrillation the diagnosis is much more likely to be embolic.

EXAMINATION

This can be remembered by the five Ps: Pain, Pallor, Pulselessness, Paraesthesia and Paralysis.

The remainder of the clinical examination is concerned with assessing the blood supply to the asymptomatic limb and determining whether there is a possible source of embolus.

Chronic occlusive arterial disease ★★★★

This is the most common type of vascular patient you will encounter in examinations. Pain is the predominant symptom and takes one of two forms:

1. Intermittent claudication: pain on exertion
2. Rest pain: continuous discomfort.

Surgical pathology Occlusive arterial disease is defined as narrowing or complete blockage of major blood vessels, usually as a result of atheroma. With respect to the lower limb, the two most common sites of occlusion are the aortoiliac region and the superficial femoral artery in the thigh. In most patients a careful history and clinical examination will determine the site of occlusion prior to radiological investigations.

HISTORY

Intermittent claudication ★★★★

Intermittent claudication is typically a cramp-like discomfort precipitated by exertion and relieved by rest. It may be unilateral or bilateral. Blood flow to the limb is adequate for tissue demands at rest, but the arterial disease prevents the increase in oxygen delivery necessary for the metabolic demands of exercise.

The history should elicit the following:

1. The site of discomfort. Patients with superficial femoral artery occlusion experience calf muscle claudication. When the aortoiliac segment is involved the patient will also experience buttock claudication, owing to the blood flow to the gluteal muscles (internal iliacs) being impaired.
2. The claudication distance, i.e. how far the patient has to walk on a level surface to precipitate pain.
3. Whether the claudication distance is progressive, static or regressive.
4. Whether the patient's symptoms interfere with their lifestyle, in terms of either work or social activities.
5. Smoking history.
6. General health, particularly with respect to cardiorespiratory disease.

Rest pain ★★★

Whereas intermittent claudication is a relatively benign condition with a low incidence of progression to amputation, rest pain is an aggressive condition with a high rate of limb loss. Many of these patients will already have had surgical or radiological intervention.

The pain is frequently described as gnawing or boring, and is often worse in bed at night. Typically patients learn to get some relief by hanging the affected limb over the edge of the bed.

Smoking history and other symptoms of cardiovascular disease (myocardial, cerebrovascular) are important. Analgesic requirements should also be assessed.

EXAMINATION

Although the following describes the examination of the legs, it cannot be divorced from examination of the entire patient. In particular, the whole cardiovascular system should receive attention.

Inspection

1. Are there any signs of ischaemia (pallor, dry scaly skin, gangrene, ulcers, nail changes, hair loss, muscle wasting etc.)? If so, is there any associated infection (cellulitis etc.)?
2. Are there any scars suggesting previous arterial surgery?
3. Does the affected limb blanche on elevation (Buerger's test)? An affected limb will also regain its colour more slowly when placed back in the horizontal position, and will often become congested and cyanosed when placed over the edge of the bed.
4. What is the state of venous filling? Venous guttering on elevation signifies impaired blood flow.

Palpation

1. Are there any discernible temperature differences between the two limbs?
2. Is there any muscle tenderness (a sign of critical muscle ischaemia)?
3. What pulses are palpable and what is their character? Compare and contrast the femoral, popliteal, posterior tibial and dorsalis pedis pulses on each side.

Auscultation

1. Listen for bruits over the major vessels. A systolic bruit indicates a stenosis, either at or above the point where the stethoscope is positioned.

FACTFILE

1. Landmarks for palpation of the lower limb pulses are as follows:

   (a) *Femoral:* The external iliac artery continues as the common femoral artery where it passes behind the inguinal ligament. The surface marking for this is the midinguinal point, which is half-way between the pubic symphysis and the anterior superior iliac spine.

   (b) *Popliteal:* Undoubtedly, the popliteal pulse is the one that poses the greatest problem. The most common error is to feel for it too high up in the popliteal fossa, where the thick fascia behind the knee joint masks it. The popliteal pulse should be felt at the level of the tibial tuberosity, where the artery lies close to bone between the two heads of the gastrocnemius muscle. The leg must be partially flexed but relaxed.

   (c) *Posterior tibial:* Immediately posterior to the medial malleolus.

   (d) *Dorsalis pedis:* On the dorsum of the foot immediately lateral to the tendon of extensor hallucis longus.   *(Cont'd)*

---

2. Investigations

(a) The ankle brachial pressure index (ABPI) is useful in patients in whom there is doubt as to whether leg pain is related to vascular disease. With the patient lying supine the systolic blood pressure is measured in the brachial and posterior tibial arteries. In a normal subject who is lying supine this ratio will be 1, and any figure under 1 is suggestive of impairment of the arterial supply to the lower limb. In general terms the ratio will be less than 0.7 in claudicants and less than 0.5 in patients with rest pain.

(b) Treadmill walking tests combined with measurement of ankle pressures are useful in making a functional assessment of the severity of disease in claudicants. This investigation can also determine whether a patient's exercise tolerance is truly impaired by claudication, as opposed to effort dyspnoea or angina.

(c) Colour flow Doppler ultrasound can assess stenoses and identify and measure the length of occlusions in larger vessels (common femoral, superficial femoral, origin of the profunda femoris and popliteal arteries).

(d) Arteriography is the gold standard investigation and is normally carried out by the Seldinger technique via one of the femoral arteries. Compared with the other investigations, however, it is an invasive procedure and is not without risk (haemorrhage, false aneurysm formation, rupture of atheromatous plaques with acute vessel occlusion or distal embolization, anaphylactic reactions to contrast media etc.) In general terms, therefore, it is reserved for patients being prepared for surgery.

3. Treatment

The majority of patients with intermittent claudication require no specific treatment. Most will improve if they stop smoking and exercise as much as possible. Intervention is reserved for patients with worsening disease, or those in whom the *(Cont'd)*

claudication distance is significantly affecting their life. Rest
pain, however, represents limb threat and justifies aggressive
management in an attempt to delay or avoid the need for
amputation. There are two principal forms of treatment:
(a) Percutaneous transluminal angioplasty (PTA)
(b) Bypass grafting. The most common grafts performed are a
bifurcation (or aortobifemoral graft) for aortoiliac disease
and a femoroproximal popliteal graft for superficial
femoral artery occlusion.
4. Prevention of reocclusion
Patency rates following PTA or grafting are significantly
improved if the patient refrains from smoking. Antiplatelet
drugs such as aspirin or dipyridamole also improve the
long-term results. Success rates are much lower following
surgery for rest pain than in claudicants.

DISCUSSION POINT

1. Should persistent smokers be offered treatment for
peripheral vascular disease?

X-RAYS ★★★

You may be asked to look at X-rays relevant to a particular
patient at any stage of a clinical examination. In addition, a
radiological station is not uncommonly used in objective
structured clinical examinations (OSCE type) or to fill in
time towards the end of a conventional clinical examination.

The following comprises a list of some of the more
commonly used films. As a general principle, make sure you
let the examiners know what the investigation is before
drawing attention to any abnormality you think is apparent.
Remember that if you look at the X-ray and do not recognize
the exact type of examination you should still describe it, for

example 'This is a film of the abdomen'. If you do not recognize anything but see contrast medium, the film may be from fluoroscopic examination so say if you think this.

Barium enema ★★★★

Usually this will be a double-contrast examination: the colon is distended with air and there is a thin coat of barium on the mucosa. The radiologist's catheter may be visible in the rectum. Usually there will be an obvious abnormality: either the typical apple-core stricture of a colonic carcinoma or a 'saw-tooth' pattern, most marked in the sigmoid, indicating diverticular disease.

Pneumoperitoneum ★★★★

The relevant film will usually be an erect chest X-ray rather than an abdominal film. Look for a lucent shadow below the diaphragm, usually most noticeable on the right. The most common causes of pneumoperitoneum are perforation of a gastric or duodenal ulcer, or perforated sigmoid diverticular disease or a postoperative film.

Intestinal obstruction ★★★★

In many instances you will be given two films, a plain (i.e. no contrast) erect and a plain supine film of the abdomen. The radiological signs of obstruction are dilated bowel loops (often most apparent on the supine film) and fluid levels (only seen on the erect film). You will be expected to know the radiological differences between small and large bowel obstruction, as follows:

- **Position** The large bowel (with the exception of the transverse colon) is situated peripherally, whereas the small bowel sits in the centre of the abdomen. Distal small bowel obstruction is often described as a ladder pattern extending from the right iliac fossa up to the left upper quadrant.

- **Calibre** The colon is broader than the small bowel.
- **Identifying features** The most important distinguishing radiological features between small and large bowel are the presence of plicae circulares or linea semilunaris in the former and haustrae in the latter. The plicae circulares characteristic of small bowel cross the full width of the bowel lumen, whereas colonic haustrae appear as indentations which do not extend right across the bowel.

You will be expected to know the common causes of intestinal obstruction, as follows:

- Small bowel obstruction: adhesions, herniae, caecal carcinoma
- Large bowel obstruction: colonic carcinoma until proven otherwise.

Beware the occasional film of distal small bowel obstruction in which the biliary tree in the right upper quadrant is outlined by gas – these appearances are classic of a gallstone ileus.

Endoscopic retrograde cholangiopancreatography (ERCP) ★★★

The giveaway here is that the endoscope will almost always appear on the film, with a fine catheter containing contrast extending from its tip. In most circumstances the abnormality will be gross, e.g. a markedly dilated common bile duct containing numerous gallstones.

Pneumothorax ★★★

Here you will be given a chest X-ray which may be marked 'expiration', as this shows up a small pneumothorax more readily. Usually, however, the pneumothorax will be large, i.e. complete absence of lung markings on one side of the chest, perhaps with mediastinal shift to the other side suggestive of a tension pneumothorax (i.e. cardiac and tracheal shadows deviated). Remember that a small pneumothorax is one of the more common 'missed' abnormalities in what is thought to be a normal chest film.

IVP films ★★

This investigation can be identified by the fact that there will be contrast in one or both of the renal pelves, and/or the ureters and bladder. Usually there will also be a time marked on the film (e.g. 10 min), indicating the time interval between the contrast being injected intravenously and the film being taken. The abnormality will usually be either complete absence of a renal tract outline on one side, indicating non-function, or a dilated ureter and renal pelvis, suggestive of an obstructing ureteric calculus.

ANEURYSMAL ARTERIAL DISEASE ★★

DEFINITIONS

An aneurysm is an abnormal dilatation associated with an artery. They can be classified as:

- **True ★★★** These comprise all layers of the vessel wall and can be saccular or fusiform in shape.
- **False ★★** Here an abnormal sac communicates with the lumen of the vessel.
- **Dissecting ★** In this instance a breach in the intima of the vessel allows the pressure of the blood flow to dissect the layers of the vessel wall, creating a second channel which may rupture back into the lumen more distally or externally.

PATHOLOGY

Aneurysms may be:

- Congenital, e.g. berry aneurysms on the circle of Willis.
- Degenerative. This is the most common type and is associated with atheromatous disease.

- Inflammatory. Infection may or may not be present and any vessel may be affected. The best-known examples are syphilitic aneurysms of the thoracic aorta and mycotic aneurysms of subacute bacterial endocarditis.
- Traumatic. Trauma (iatrogenic or otherwise) can lead to damage or weakening of a vessel wall and the creation of either a true or a false aneurysm.

HISTORY

The only type of aneurysm you are likely to encounter in the clinical examination is one affecting the abdominal aorta. Patients with such an aneurysm may well be asymptomatic, and indeed the presence of an aneurysm may have been an incidental finding on admission for some other purpose. Alternatively, some patients experience intermittent back and/or abdominal pain. More importantly, the history should focus on the general health of the patient, particularly with respect to cardiovascular risk factors.

EXAMINATION

Abdominal aortic aneurysms are palpable in the epigastrium (the aorta bifurcates just above the level of the umbilicus). It is a characteristic feature of an aneurysm that the pulsation is expansile, and it is this feature that differentiates an aneurysm from transmitted pulsation, for example, through, a gastric mass.

In estimating the size of the aneurysm the hands are brought together from either side of the abdomen until the expansile pulsation is felt. One to two centimetres usually have to be deducted from this measured pulsation to allow for abdominal wall fat.

As for occlusive arterial disease, the entire cardiovascular system, and in particular distal pulses, should be assessed.

Investigations

1. X-rays. Calcification within the vessel wall may be seen on a plain abdominal radiograph.
2. Ultrasound. This allows accurate measurements to be made of the aneurysm's size and will usually identify the upper and lower limits.
3. Angiography. This is rarely required, but occasionally may be necessary to determine the relationship of the upper extent of the aneurysm to the renal arteries prior to surgery.

TREATMENT

This will be determined by:

1. The size of the aneurysm. Asymptomatic aneurysms of less than 5 cm diameter may be managed conservatively by regular ultrasound and clinical examination.
2. The general health of the patient. The majority of patients with degenerative aortic aneurysms will have generalized arterial disease and are at risk of myocardial or cerebral infarction. In addition, as most of these patients are smokers, chronic chest disease is common.
3. The patient's age. This is not as important as general health but, although surgeons vary, most will place an upper limit on the age at which they are prepared to operate.

RENAL FAILURE (surgical aspects) ★★

Occasionally patients from the renal unit may be used in surgical examinations. Many of them will have undergone multiple surgical procedures, some of which are peculiar to haemodialysis or peritoneal dialysis.

DEFINITIONS

Tenckhoff catheter ★★★
A catheter which is inserted into the peritoneal cavity for the purposes of peritoneal dialysis.

Arteriovenous fistula ★★★
A surgically created communication between an artery and a vein, which is required for haemodialysis. The procedure usually involves anastomosing the radial artery to the cephalic vein on the anterior aspect of the distal forearm.

Vein loop ★★★
This is an alternative to creating a fistula for vessel access for haemodialysis, and may be necessary when previous fistulae have failed. Most commonly the upper long saphenous vein is taken from the leg, tunnelled in the anterior aspect of the forearm and anastomosed to the brachial artery and cephalic vein at the level of the elbow.

Gore-tex loop ★★★
The principle of this is identical to the vein loop, except that a prosthetic graft is used instead of vein. This may be necessary if the saphenous veins have previously been removed (varicose vein surgery or previous vascular access procedures) or are unsuitable.

EXAMINATION

Be alert to the possibility of renal failure patients participating in examinations. Those on regular dialysis will usually appear anaemic ('normal' haemoglobins for renal failure patients may be 7–9 g/dl), and tend to have multiple scars on their forearms and/or abdomen. Patients with functioning transplants are usually of a more normal colour but frequently appear mildly Cushingoid, owing to their long-standing immunosuppression. Arteriovenous fistulae will be evident as dilated superficial vessels on the distal forearm (the 'arterialized' vein). If functioning, there will be a palpable thrill and a bruit will be heard if a stethoscope is placed over it. The surgical scar will usually be sited over the anterior and lateral aspects of the distal forearm, signifying the approach to the radial artery. Vein loops and Gore-tex loops are anastomosed to the brachial artery and cephalic veins at the level of the elbow, and there will be scars at this level. The loop is tunnelled subcutaneously so that the apex lies on the anterior aspect of the forearm, approximately half-way between the elbow and the wrist, where there will usually be a further small scar. Function is indicated by a palpable pulse, a thrill and an audible bruit. If the patient has a vein loop there will be a long scar along the anteromedial thigh through which the upper long saphenous vein has been harvested. Tenckhoff catheters are usually made of opaque silicone and pass through the abdominal wall a few centimetres to one side of a small laparotomy incision (either midline or paramedian).

Palpable abdominal abnormalities in renal patients may include polycystic kidneys (very large renal masses) or a transplanted kidney. The latter is felt in one or other iliac fossa underlying a curved scar extending from above the anterior superior iliac spine towards the midline just above the pubic symphysis.

Remember that renal failure patients commonly have conditions of surgical interest which may be brought to your attention. Most notably, diabetes and peripheral vascular disease are common.

AN A–Z IN SURGERY

QUESTIONS

ABDOMINOPERINEAL RESECTION

A1 What is this procedure and what condition is it most commonly used to treat?

ACHALASIA

A2 What is achalasia and how might it present?

AMAUROSIS FUGAX

A3 What is meant by this term and what is its significance?

AORTIC ANEURYSM

A4 Where do most aortic aneurysms occur, what is their aetiology, and how may they present?

APPENDICITIS

A5 What are the clinical features of appendicitis?

BASAL CELL CARCINOMA

B1 Where does this condition commonly occur and what individuals are at greatest risk?

BLOOD

B2 What blood tests should be taken before embarking on any form of surgical procedure or invasive investigation in a jaundiced patient?

BREAST CANCER

B3 What risk factors are recognized for breast cancer and how can they be reduced?

BREAST LUMPS

B4 What are the common causes of breast lumps in women in the reproductive age group?

BUERGER'S TEST

B5 What is this test for and how is it performed?

BURNS

B6 What is the rule of nines?

CELLULITIS

C1 What is this condition and how would you treat it?

CHOLANGITIS

C2 What are the typical symptoms and signs of acute cholangitis?

COLON CANCER

C3 What risk factors are recognized for colonic cancer?

COURVOISIER'S LAW

C4 What does this state and what is its significance?

CROHN'S DISEASE

C5 What surgical complications of Crohn's disease might make laparotomy necessary?

DIVERTICULAR DISEASE

D1 How might diverticular disease present acutely?

DUKES' CLASSIFICATION

D2 Outline Dukes' classification and its prognostic significance.

DUODENAL ULCERS

D3 What features in symptomatic enquiry are said to suggest a duodenal rather than a gastric ulcer, and is the distinction reliable?

D4 What important aetiological factor for duodenal ulcer disease has emerged in recent years?

DUPUYTREN'S CONTRACTURE

D5 What is this condition?

EMBOLISM

E1 Define this term and give an example.

ERCP

E2 What do these initials stand for? Give an indication for the use of the technique.

EVENING PRIMROSE OIL

E3 Why should oil of evening primrose improve benign breast disease?

EXTRADURAL HAEMORRHAGE

E4 Describe the typical injury which leads to this condition.

FAMILIAL ADENOMATOUS POLYPOSIS (FAP)

F1 What are the characteristics and importance of this condition?

FEMORAL ARTERY

F2 What is the surface marking of the femoral artery, and what is the relationship of the femoral nerve and femoral vein to it?

FLAIL CHEST

F3 What is this condition and how is it treated?

FRACTURES

F4 What are the causes of non-union in a case of fractured head of femur?

GALLSTONE ILEUS

G1 What is this condition and what radiological signs lend their support to the diagnosis?

GASTRIC CANCER

G2 What do you know about the epidemiology of gastric cancer?

GREY TURNER'S SIGN

G3 What is this sign and what is its significance?

GYNAECOMASTIA

G4 What is gynaecomastia and with what conditions may it be associated?

HAEMATEMESIS

H1 What are the causes of haematemesis, and how should these cases be investigated?

HAEMATURIA

H2 What are the common causes of macroscopic haematuria and how would you investigate a patient with this condition?

HAEMOPTYSIS

H3 What is the significance of haemoptysis combined with the sudden onset of pleuritic chest pain and breathlessness in a 70-year-old patient 10 days following major intra-abdominal surgery for malignant disease?

HERNIA

H4 What is meant by the term 'hernia' and what types do you know?

HYDROCOELE

H5 What is a hydrocoele and how would you distinguish it from other swellings in that area?

ILEOSTOMY

I1 How can you distinguish an ileostomy from a colostomy?

INTERMITTENT CLAUDICATION

I2 How does the history give you an indication of the level of arterial occlusion?

INTESTINAL OBSTRUCTION

I3   What radiological features distinguish small bowel from large bowel obstruction?

IRRITABLE BOWEL SYNDROME (IBS)

I4   How is IBS diagnosed?

JAUNDICE

J1   What causes of obstructive jaundice do you know?

KELOID

K1   What is meant by this term?

KIDNEY

K2   What congenital abnormalities of the kidneys do you know of?

K3   What other associated problems might there be and how are they managed?

KILLIAN'S DEHISCENCE

K4   Where would you find this?

KRUKENBERG TUMOUR

K5   What is meant by this term?

LEG ULCERS

L1   What are the causes of leg ulcers?

L2   What long-term effects are seen in cases of varicose ulcers?

LONG SAPHENOUS VEIN

L3   Describe the course of the long saphenous vein.

LYMPHADENOPATHY

L4   What are the causes of lymph node enlargement?

LYMPHOEDEMA

L5   What is lymphoedema?

MALLORY–WEISS SYNDROME

M1   What is Mallory–Weiss syndrome?

MARJOLIN'S ULCER

M2   What is this condition?

MECKEL'S DIVERTICULUM

M3   What are the characteristics of a Meckel's diverticulum?

MELAENA

M4   What is melaena and what does it signify?

MELANOMA

M5   What are signs of malignant change in a pigmented lesion?

M6   How are cases of malignant melanoma best managed?

NAILS

N1   How are ingrowing toenails managed?

NECROTIZING FASCIITIS

N2   How common is necrotizing fasciitis and what procedures may it complicate?

NERVES

N3   What is the typical appearance of the hand if the ulnar nerve is transected at the elbow?

NIPPLE DISCHARGE

N4   What factors are important in assessing a patient with nipple discharge in terms of assessing the need for surgery?

NUTRITION

N5   What are some of the indications for total parenteral nutrition (TPN)?

ODDI

O1   Where is the sphincter of Oddi?

OESOPHAGEAL VARICES

O2 What are the causes of oesophageal varices and how do they present?

OSGOOD—SCHLATTER'S DISEASE

O3 What is this condition?

PANCREATITIS

P1 How would you assess the severity of an attack of acute pancreatitis?

PEUTZ—JEGHER SYNDROME?

P2 What is Peutz—Jegher syndrome?

PNEUMOTHORAX

P3 How would you recognize a tension pneumothorax and how would you treat it?

PYLORIC STENOSIS

P4 At what age does congenital pyloric obstruction present?

QUINSY

Q1 What is meant by the term quinsy and how is this condition treated?

RECTAL EXAMINATION

R1 What are the indications for a rectal examination?

SENGSTAKEN TUBE

S1 What is this and what is it used for?

SPLENECTOMY

S2 What are the indications for splenectomy and what long-term complications may result?

S3 How might these be reduced?

TESTIS

T1 What are the clinical features of torsion of the testis?

T2 What is the differential diagnosis?

THROMBOEMBOLISM

T3 How can you reduce the risk of deep venous thrombosis and pulmonary thromboembolism following major abdominal surgery?

ULCERATIVE COLITIS

U1 What is the incidence of colonic cancer in patients with ulcerative colitis?

U2 What factors influence the site of a stoma in such patients?

VAGOTOMY

V1 What are some of the sequelae of truncal vagotomy for peptic ulcer disease?

VARICOCOELE

V2 What is a varicocoele?

VARICOSE VEINS

V3 What options are available for the treatment of lower limb varices?

WILM'S TUMOUR

W1 What is the 5-year survival rate for Wilm's tumour presenting below the age of 3?

WOUND DEHISCENCE

W2 What factors predispose to dehiscence of an abdominal wound in the postoperative period?

X-RAYS

X1 What percentage of gallstones are radiologically obvious in a plain X-ray of the abdomen? What percentage of kidney stones are radiologically obvious in a plain X-ray of the abdomen?

ZADIK'S OPERATION

Z1 What condition is this procedure used to treat?

ZOLLINGER–ELLISON SYNDROME

Z2   What is this?

Z-PLASTY?

Z3   What is meant by this term?

ANSWERS

A1   Excision of the entire rectum, anal canal and anus, usually for carcinoma of the lower rectum.

A2   Failure of relaxation of the lower end of the oesophagus, leading to progressive dilatation and tortuosity of the oesophagus. Dysphagia, regurgitation and aspiration are the symptoms.

A3   Sudden but transient unilateral loss of vision, which may be secondary to embolization from an ulcerated atheromatous plaque at the carotid bifurcation. In suitable cases surgery may reduce the risk of subsequent stroke.

A4   The most common site is the abdominal aorta below the origin of the renal arteries. Such aneurysms are secondary to atheromatous disease, and frequently are discovered as an asymptomatic pulsatile mass in the upper abdomen during routine clinical examination. They may cause back pain and can present as an emergency, with sudden abdominal pain and circulatory collapse secondary to their rupture.

A5   Periumbilical colicky pain moving to the right iliac fossa as a continuous pain. Nausea, anorexia and vomiting are common features.

B1   These tumours are most frequently seen on the forehead and upper part of the face in elderly individuals.

Fair-skinned people constantly exposed to strong sunlight are at greatest risk. Although locally invasive, the tumour rarely metastasizes.

B2 Hepatitis screen and coagulation screen.

B3 Family history, parity and breastfeeding practice all play a role. The role of HRT remains controversial, at least among gynaecologists. Promoting breastfeeding should reduce the risks.

B4 Fibroadenoma, carcinoma, breast cysts, fat necrosis, abscess.

B5 This is a test for arterial insufficiency of the lower limb. The patient's legs are raised to 45° from the horizontal and if the arterial supply is defective the distal limb will become pale, with guttering of the veins on the dorsum of the foot. If the legs are then hung over the edge of the bed, within a few moments they will take on a ruddy cyanotic appearance.

B6 This is a method to describe the surface area of the body and is used to estimate the area affected by burns. Thus, each arm is considered as 9%, 9% for the head and neck, 9×2 i.e. 18% for each leg and for the front of the trunk, and also for the back of the trunk. The perineum is considered as 1%.

C1 Cellulitis is characterized by spreading inflammation in the subcutaneous plane, and is usually caused by beta-haemolytic streptococcal infection. Treatment comprises immobilization, elevation if a limb is the affected part, and treatment with benzylpenicillin.

C2 This condition is characterized by Charcot's triad: high fever, rigors and jaundice. Typically the condition is caused by impacted stones in the common bile duct.

C3   Family history, benign polyps, long-standing inflammatory bowel disease.

C4   The law states that if in the presence of obstructive jaundice the gallbladder is palpable then the obstruction is unlikely to be due to stones. The implication is that carcinoma of the head of the pancreas must be suspected, as a diseased gallbladder giving rise to gallstones would be less likely to distend than a normal viscus. The law is of course not absolute, as the two pathologies can coexist.

C5   Perforation, obstruction, fistula formation, bleeding.

D1   Perforation, bleeding, occasionally obstruction.

D2   Dukes originally described three stages to classify the extent of spread of rectal carcinoma. Since then a fourth stage has been added, and it is commonly applied to large bowel cancer at all sites. The stages are:

    A: Tumour confined to the rectal wall: 5-year survival approximately 95%

    B: Tumour penetrated the rectal wall: 5-year survival approximately 70%

    C: Spread to the regional lymph nodes: 5-year survival approximately 30%

    D: Distant metastases: 5-year survival less than 5%.

D3   Hunger pain and relief by food and antacids suggest duodenal rather than gastric ulcer. These are not clinically reliable.

D4   Infection with *Helicobacter pylori*, which leads to increased gastrin secretion and increased sensitivity of the gastric parietal cells to gastrin, resulting in increased acid secretion.

D5 Dupuytren's contracture is characterized by thickening and foreshortening of the palmar aponeurosis and this gives rise to flexion contractures of the fingers. The aetiology is uncertain, but there is an increased incidence in association with alcohol-induced chronic liver disease.

E1 The transfer of abnormal material through the bloodstream and its impaction in a smaller vessel more distally. The clinical symptoms and signs will be determined by the affected vascular tree, but examples include stroke (from the heart in atrial fibrillation or ulcerated plaques at the carotid bifurcation), pulmonary thromboembolism (detachment of clot, usually from the proximal leg or pelvic veins) or peripheral arterial embolism (from the heart or from atheromatous plaques more proximal in the arterial tree). The latter will be characterized by the six Ps: pain, pallor, pulselessness, paralysis, paraesthesia, and perishing with cold.

E2 Endoscopic retrograde cholangiopancreatography. ERCP can be a diagnostic technique to establish the cause of obstructive jaundice, a dilated biliary tree, and for the investigation of pancreatic disease, or a therapeutic procedure, as in extraction of common bile duct stones and stenting of malignant bile duct obstruction.

E3 Gammolenic acid contained in evening primrose oil is an essential fatty acid which is a precursor in prostaglandin metabolism, which is effective in mastalgia but requires treatment for between 8 and 12 weeks to be effective.

E4 Extradural haemorrhage occurs following an injury to the side of the head, which can be relatively trivial. Typically there is a fracture of the temporal bone which results in a tear to the middle meningeal artery. Urgent neurosurgical referral is required.

F1 FAP is characterized by the development of multiple polyps through the large bowel which, if left untreated, will eventually become carcinomatous. It is transmitted by autosomal dominant inheritance and the polyps usually develop in late childhood or early adult life. Prevention of carcinoma necessitates total colectomy.

F2 The external iliac artery passes behind the inguinal ligament to become the femoral artery at the midinguinal point, i.e. midway between the anterior superior iliac spine and the pubic symphisis. The vein lies on its medial side and the nerve is lateral to it.

F3 A flail chest is characterized by paradoxical movement of part of the chest wall, i.e. the affected part is drawn in on inspiration. It occurs when multiple ribs are fractured at both ends. When large there can be marked hypoxia, owing to failure of ventilation of the underlying lung and cardiovascular impairment. Mild cases require oxygen therapy, analgesia and physiotherapy, but severe cases may require positive pressure ventilation.

F4 Avascular necrosis, infection, pathology, e.g. sarcoma, loss of apposition, interposition of soft tissue.

G1 Small bowel obstruction secondary to a large gallstone passing through a fistulous connection between the gallbladder and duodenum and impacting in the terminal ileum. Radiological signs include the typical features of small bowel obstruction combined with air in the biliary tree as a result of the cholecystoduodenal fistula.

G2 Widespread geographical variation, with Japan having a particularly high incidence. High intake of dietary nitrate. Smoked fish is implicated. Pernicious anaemia, atrophic gastritis and previous gastric ulcer.

G3   Bluish discoloration in the flanks secondary to extravasation of blood from haemorrhagic pancreatitis.

G4   Enlargement of the male breast, which may be precipitated by drugs (cimetidine, digoxin) or associated with some other illness (chronic liver disease or some testicular tumours). Gynaecomastia is also not uncommon at puberty, and most cases will settle spontaneously.

H1   Ulcer, (gastric or duodenal), oesophagitis, varices, erosions, Mallory–Weiss tear. Endoscopy is the investigation of choice.

H2   Important renal tract causes include trauma, kidney or bladder tumours, calculus disease, prostatic hypertrophy or prostatic carcinoma. In the absence of a systemic cause investigation will include cystoscopy and an intravenous urogram. Haematuria may also be secondary to systemic disease, such as a bleeding disorder or anticoagulant therapy.

H3   The symptom combination and timescale from surgery are classic of pulmonary thromboembolism. Urgent anticoagulation and further investigation are required to confirm the diagnosis.

H4   Protrusion of whole or part of a viscus through an opening in the wall of the cavity in which it is normally contained. External herniae include inguinal, femoral, paraumbilical, epigastric, incisional, obturator and spigelian.

H5   A collection of fluid in the tunica vaginalis in the scrotum. It can be distinguished from an inguinoscrotal hernia by the fact that you can get your fingers above it and by its characteristic transillumination. Epidydimal cysts may also transilluminate, but they lie above and posterior to the testis, whereas a hydrocoele is anterior and cannot be separated from the testis.

I1 An ileostomy will usually be sited in the right iliac fossa, whereas a colostomy will more often be encountered on the left side of the abdomen. In addition, the contents of an ileostomy bag will be fluid-like and often bile stained. Most importantly, however, an ileostomy will be everted to form a spout whereas a colostomy will tend to be almost flush with the skin.

I2 The two common sites affected are either the aortoiliac segment of the arterial tree or the superficial femoral artery. If the former is occluded the patient will suffer buttock claudication, whereas superficial femoral artery disease presents as calf claudication.

I3 Calibre, the central position of the small bowel as compared with the more peripherally sited colon, and the presence of plicae circulares extending the full width of the small bowel.

I4 By exclusion of other causes of the major symptoms, i.e. colicky abdominal pain, diarrhoea, change in bowel habit and bloatedness.

J1 Gallstones, cancer of head of pancreas, cholangiocarcinoma, benign strictures.

K1 A form of wound healing characterized by the production of excessive amounts of dense hyalinised fibrous tissue which results in a raised and broadened scar.

K2 Pelvic kidney, horseshoe kidneys, ureteric duplication, vascular abnormalities.

K3 Vesicoureteric reflux and recurrent urinary tract infection are the commonest complications of congenital renal abnormality.

K4 At the back of the pharynx. This is the defect between the two parts of the inferior constrictor of the pharynx, where a pharyngeal pouch develops.

K5 Ovarian metastases from carcinoma of the stomach (usually signet ring) as a result of transperitoneal spread.

L1 Arterial insufficiency and venous stasis.

L2 Chiefly, Marjolin's ulcer.

L3 The long saphenous vein arises from the dorsal venous arch of the foot, passes anterior to the medial malleolus at the ankle, up the medial side of the leg and knee to drain into the femoral vein via the fossa ovalis.

L4 Reactive, i.e. following infection. Pathological, i.e. malignancy.

L5 Pitting oedema owing to the accumulation of protein-rich fluid in the tissues. It results from lymphatic obstruction, which can be primary or secondary, for example lymphoedema of the arm following axillary surgery for breast cancer.

M1 A tear at the oesophagogastric junction which gives rise to upper gastrointestinal tract bleeding. It occurs following prolonged vomiting or retching.

M2 Squamous carcinoma developing at the edge of a long-standing skin ulcer secondary to chronic irritation.

M3 A Meckel's diverticulum lies on the antimesenteric border of the terminal ileum and is a remnant of the vitellointestinal duct. It occurs in approximately 2% of the population, within 2 feet of the caecum, and is approximately 2 inches in length. Most are asymptomatic but occasionally they can become inflamed.

M4 Offensive tarry black stools secondary to the action of digestive enzymes on blood in the lumen of the upper gastrointestinal tract. It therefore signifies upper gastrointestinal tract bleeding, although on occasions the source of blood loss can be as distal as the caecum.

M5   Increase in size, changes in pigmentation, haemorrhage, ulceration and satellite lesions.

M6   This depends on the depth of invasion, but usually involves wide local excision and may require block dissection of affected lymph nodes. Chemotherapy may also be required, but radiotherapy is only given as a palliative.

N1   Treatment may be conservative, involving chiropodists, or surgical by simple avulsion with or without nailbed ablation.

N2   The incidence is unknown owing to variation in reporting rates. It most frequently follows perineal and scrotal trauma, surgery, particularly if infected, or involving a hollow viscus.

N3   As the intrinsic muscles are paralysed, claw hand develops owing to the unopposed action of the long finger flexors and extensors.

N4   Discharge which is bloodstained and coming from a single duct should always be taken seriously, as this may indicate an underlying intraduct papilloma or carcinoma. Bilateral multiduct discharge devoid of blood staining, on the other hand, is most probably due to the benign condition duct ectasia.

N5   Enteral nutrition via the gastrointestinal tract is the preferred method of feeding whenever possible, but TPN may be necessary on occasions. These include instances where one cannot obtain easy access to the gut, for example in oesophageal obstruction; when the gut is not functioning as in prolonged ileus; when one wishes to deliberately rest the gut; or when it is impossible to get sufficient nutrition into the body, as in short gut syndrome and severe burns.

O1   At the lower end of the common bile duct.

O2   These varices are associated with portal hypertension, that is, a portal venous pressure of 20 cm H_2O or greater. They present as acute major upper gastrointestinal haemorrhage or chronic blood loss.

O3   Apophysitis of the tibial tubercle, which results in the tubercle becoming enlarged and painful. It is most common in early teenage boys and the symptoms are aggravated by exercise.

P1   The serum amylase level is a diagnostic tool and gives no indication of the severity of the illness. This is assessed by Imrie's prognostic criteria.

P2   An autosomal dominant condition characterized by gastrointestinal tract polyposis, mucosal pigmentation and hamartomatous lesions.

P3   Rapidly progressive respiratory distress, hyper-resonance on percussion over the affected side, deviation of the trachea and apex beat away from the affected side. The affected pleural cavity must be drained urgently, if necessary by the insertion of a cannula through an intercostal space until a water seal drain is available.

P4   Usually between 3–4 weeks.

Q1   Peritonsillar abscess. It is treated by incision and drainage.

R1   Any gastrointestinal tract disease or suspicion thereof.

S1   A double-balloon tube which is used in the emergency treatment of bleeding gastro-oesophageal varices. The gastric balloon is fluid filled and pulled back against the gastro-oesophageal junction while the oesophageal balloon is inflated to a pressure of 30–40 mmHg to directly compress the oesophageal varices.

S2 Trauma. Some haematological disorders. It is no longer routinely employed to stage Hodgkin's disease. Long-term complications include infection, particularly with *Haemophilus influenzae* and *Streptococcus pneumoniae*.

S3 Vaccination against pneumococcal infection reduces risk. Emergency splenectomy should be covered with antibiotic prophylaxis. Some advocate treatment for 2 years, whereas others suggest lifelong treatment.

T1 Sudden onset of low abdominal and testicular pain, with a tender swollen testis and oedematous scrotum.

T2 Differential diagnosis includes epididymo-orchitis.

T3 Early mobilization, regular subcutaneous heparin, graduated lower limb compression stockings, intermittent calf compression in the operating theatre, and correction of preoperative factors in elective cases, e.g. smoking, the oral contraceptive pill.

U1 Total colitis for 10 years carries a risk of malignancy of 2%, rising to 30% at 30 years.

U2 Site of stoma is influenced by existing scars, skin folds and indication for surgery.

V1 Failure of gastric emptying (gastroparesis) and diarrhoea can be attributed directly to the vagotomy. There are a number of other potential complications associated with the accompanying drainage procedure, including dumping, anaemia and bilious vomiting.

V2 Commonly believed to be varicosities of the pampiniform plexus of veins, although in some cases the venous, dilatation may involve the cremasteric vessels. Varicocoeles are more common on the left side of the scrotum and have a characteristic 'bag of worms' feeling when the patient stands.

V3 Conservative, e.g. support tights. Surgical, e.g. sclerotherapy and high ligation of the long saphenous vein.

W1 80–90% chance of cure.

W2 Poor surgical technique, wound infection, chronic cough, conditions which impair healing, e.g. uraemia, diabetes, advanced malignant disease, severe sepsis, and certain drugs such as corticosteroids.

X1 10% of gallstones are radiologically obvious and 90% of kidney stones can be seen on X-ray.

Z1 An ingrown toenail. The procedure involves formal excision of the germinal matrix of the nail.

Z2 Excessive gastric acid secretion secondary to a gastrin-producing tumour, which is most commonly in the pancreas. Extensive duodenal ulceration develops in many cases extending distally as far as the jejunum.

Z3 A procedure using a pedicle flap, generally in plastic surgery.

GYNAECOLOGY

HISTORY AND EXAMINATION IN GYNAECOLOGY

PRESENTING THE GYNAECOLOGICAL CASE

The summary style for presenting a case is useful in gynae-cology. The principle underlying this is to give the basic information about the patient in order to fix the examiners' attention. The ability to identify the key points in the history is worth developing, and essential for clinical practice. Thus you may wish to present 'Mrs Smith, a 53-year-old insulin-dependent diabetic with postmenopausal bleeding'. This 'sets the stage' and allows the examiners to focus directly on the clinical problem. In certain cases it is appropriate to summarize and give the symptomatology in the patient's words. For example Mrs Smith might complain of 'something coming down', and because you will not have done a vaginal examination until the examiners are present you cannot present her as a case of prolapse. General examination is done as in medicine and surgery, although urine testing is often omitted.

Have as well-developed a scheme as possible for presenting abdominal findings. Even if there are no masses do not just say 'The abdomen was OK': the findings should be as comprehensively presented as in the surgical finals.

Examiners may ask you to demonstrate your technique of abdominal palpation. This is the same as described in the surgical section, although often gynaecologists do not insist on finding a seat or kneeling to be at the same level as the abdomen. The important point here is that after the standard abdominal palpation technique, gynaecologists often make a point of examining the pelvic organs abdominally with the left hand (standing on the patient's right side). You should comment generally on scars and on the presence or absence of organomegaly. Remember to check for lymphadenopathy, which is readily forgotten (including supraclavicular and cervical nodes).

A number of medical schools no longer insist on vaginal examination in the finals. However, when it is to be undertaken, it is only performed once and in the presence of the examiners. Candidates worry at length about whether to perform a speculum or digital examination first. Similarly, some people get quite worked up about how much lubricating gel to apply, if any. The rule is to use whatever technique you are accustomed to as long as you can justify your selected approach. It is worth noting, however, that the Intercollegiate Working Party of the Royal College of Obstetricians and Gynaecologists and the Royal College of Pathologists on cervical cytology screening suggest that 'lubricant may be used sparingly to facilitate the passage of the speculum but care must be taken to avoid contamination of the cervix'.

You will probably be asked at the end to summarize your history and findings, so do this. Do not repeat the whole story again: this is really annoying and wastes time. Only positive points need be mentioned at this stage. This applies when you are asked to summarize for any clinical exams.

THE CASES

CONTRACEPTION/STERILIZATION ★★★★★

Contraception is such a basic part of gynaecological practice that related topics can be introduced as part of the discussion at virtually any stage of a gynaecological examination. In terms of an actual case which might be seen in the clinical examination, however, it is much likelier that an elective admission for sterilization will be seen.

DEFINITION

Sterilization is an operation the intention of which is to produce permanent, irreversible and reliable contraception.

HISTORY

This is difficult to deal with in terms of presentation if there is no other significant history. This may be a problem for both you and the examiners to tackle. The important facets to deal with are the previous method of contraception and reasons why this is no longer acceptable.

When taking the history it is worth identifying what counselling the patient has received: for example, is she aware of failure rates, irreversibility, the possible need for laparotomy during some laparoscopic procedures, and the risk of ectopic pregnancy? It is not your function to counsel the patient, so beware of alarming her about the risks: for example, it is not universal practice to warn of the risk of ectopic pregnancy.

EXAMINATION

This is likely to be unremarkable but does not excuse the lack of a comprehensive examination. During the vaginal examination it is important to demonstrate your capacity to be efficient and thorough, as it is unlikely that there will be any significant abnormality.

FACTFILE

1. Failure rates per 100 women years, i.e. number of pregnancies per 100 women using a particular technique for 1 year:
   - Combined oral contraceptive 0.16–0.27
   - Progesterone pill 2–3
   - Intrauterine contraceptive device (second generation) 1.0–1.5
   - Diaphragm 1.9
   - Condom 3.6
   - Male sterilization 0.02
   - Female sterilization 0.13.

2. Much attention is given to the adverse effects of oral contraception, but there are a number of benefits. Among these are reductions in the risks of endometrial and ovarian cancer, and of endometriosis. Non-gynaecological benefits are a reduction in the morbidity of rheumatoid arthritis and of thyroid disorders.

3. The side-effect profile of 50 μg pills includes that of venous thrombosis and fatal thromboembolism. Impaired glucose tolerance and cholecystitis are significantly increased. These are much reduced with lower-dose preparations.

4. The side-effect profile of injectable progestogens includes erratic vaginal bleeding, which may on occasion complicate the diagnosis of pregnancy.

5. The operative mortality of female sterilization is less than 8 per 100 000 operations, but this contrasts with virtually nil for vasectomy under local anaesthesia.

DISCUSSION POINTS

1. You should be familiar with which methods of contraception are most suitable for different patients.
2. The precautions that should be observed before prescribing the oral contraceptive pill should be clearly known. You may be invited to discuss how you would manage a woman on the pill, and what observations should be made in the longer term.

MENORRHAGIA ★★★★★

DEFINITION

Heavy regular menstruation.

An alternative definition which might be introduced with benefit here is that of 'normal' menstruation, which is menstruation occurring in a cycle between 21 and 35 days, lasting between 2 and 7 days and associated with a blood loss of around 40 ml.

Dysfunctional uterine bleeding is defined as excessive menstrual loss in the absence of any clinically identified gynaecological abnormality.

Many terms are used to describe abnormalities of menstruation, such as metrorrhagia and polymenorrhoea. These are best replaced by more descriptive terms, such as irregular heavy menstruation or frequent periods. The only term which remains universally acceptable, because of the consensus about its meaning, is menorrhagia, which is in common usage. Remember that, by definition, a single epsiode of heavy vaginal bleeding cannot be called menorrhagia.

The commoner causes of excessive menstrual loss are:

- Dysfunctional uterine bleeding ★★★★★
- Pelvic inflammatory disease ★★★★
- Endometriosis (including adenomyosis) ★★★★

- Fibroid uterus ★★★★★
- Endometrial polyps ★★★
- Obesity ★★
- Anovulation ★★
- Hyper/hypothyroidism ★
- Endometrial hyperplasia/malignancy ★★
- Familial coagulation disorders ★

HISTORY

The important points are to obtain an adequate history which allows you to describe the pattern of blood loss in terms of volume and duration. A history of treatment for iron deficiency is important, as is one of clotting or flooding, indicating that the plasmin system is overwhelmed. A history of long-term oral contraceptive use is also important, as there is now a generation of women who are unaware of what a normal (i.e. non-hormonal) menstrual cycle is like. One of the results of this is that, although sterilization might be associated with changes in uterine and ovarian blood flow and menstrual loss, the commonest reason for a complaint of heavy periods following sterilization is the return of 'genuine' menstruation following cessation of pill use.

The other interesting point is that, although academics suggest that it is mandatory that a scientific method be used to estimate menstrual blood loss quantitatively, there is no relationship between actual volume of loss and the patients' symptomatology, i.e. some women with a blood loss of 35 ml will complain bitterly of heavy periods, whereas others with losses of 80 ml may not complain, or only present following a diagnosis of iron-deficiency anaemia. Nevertheless, examiners will expect a determined effort at estimating the degree of blood loss and, as above, the presence of passing clots is important. Also useful is the number of sanitary pads/tampons used.

EXAMINATION

General examination is important. You should be demonstrating that you are aware of the systemic effects and signs of anaemia. The examiners may not be particularly interested in the cardiovascular findings, but if you find a flow murmur this might be of significance. (**NB**: Do not be too clever. If there is no other clinical evidence of anaemia you might be reporting such a finding in a patient with a haemoglobin of 14 g/dl.)

On vaginal examination you should be thinking of excluding a pelvic abnormality. It is more likely however, that your patient will be undergoing investigation for dysfunctional uterine bleeding or admitted for hysterectomy or endometrial resection.

If you find an abnormality on vaginal examination think of how this ties in with the history and consider whether it is logical. For example, do not immediately suggest an intrauterine pregnancy with threatened abortion in a 45-year-old with regular heavy menses and a bulky uterus. (Adenomyosis or multiple small fibroids are more likely, and the former is only diagnosed by pathological examination of the uterus.)

FACTFILE

1. The average menstrual blood loss in women not receiving hormonal contraception is 33 ml. The 95th centile for menstrual loss is 76 ml.

2. Excessive menses is the commonest cause of anaemia in women in the reproductive age group in the UK.

3. Two-thirds of women with blood loss of 80 ml or more are anaemic.

4. Although diagnostic curettage is performed to exclude more significant contributory disease, polyps are found in only 2% of D&C specimens and, in women below the age of 36, the incidence of endometrial cancer is 1 per 100 000.

CHRONIC PELVIC PAIN ★★★★

DEFINITION

There is no standard definition of chronic pelvic pain, although increasingly some clinicians use the phrase to describe pelvic pain when obvious causes such as endometriosis and pelvic inflammatory disease have been excluded. Others use the term to describe the constellation of clinical features that are ascribed to pelvic congestion. There has been a recent recommendation to use the term PPWOP, i.e. pelvic pain without pathology. This has absolutely nothing to commend it.

HISTORY

Often the patient will have been admitted for laparoscopy, so that when you see her the common causes of pelvic pain will not necessarily have been excluded. There may be a history of previous laparoscopy sufficiently in the distant past to make the clinician repeat it, even if it was negative at the time in terms of finding a cause. Previous laparotomy including appendicectomy is worthy of note, and the patient may be able to say if the appendix was actually diseased when removed. The specific features said to be associated with the pelvic congestion type of chronic pelvic pain are of premenstrual ache and 'heaviness' in the pelvis. There is no dyspareunia as such, but typically there is pelvic pain the morning after intercourse.

One of the features of so-called pelvic congestion syndrome is the high incidence of pre-existing psychological upset, and this has been commonly described, but you will be unlikely to elicit such a history under the conditions of the examination, though a history of social problems and marital disharmony is commonplace.

EXAMINATION

This will usually be unrewarding, but remember to identify any scars, including laparoscopy scars, as some women will forget to mention previous investigations, particularly if the findings were negative. It can be quite embarrassing if the examiner points out the laparoscopy scar which he knows about from the patient's notes but which you had missed.

The speculum and vaginal examinations are directed at excluding pelvic disease such as endometriosis, and even if you elicit tenderness which you suspect has a psychological element to it, it is wrong to assume that the examiner will agree with you. Excluding chronic pelvic inflammatory disease or endometriosis will seem more relevant to him or her.

FACTFILE

1. There are no long-term follow-up data on women who have undergone 'negative laparoscopy' in the evaluation of their chronic pelvic pain.
2. Uterine and ovarian varices have been demonstrated in a high proportion of cases of chronic pelvic pain, but there are no control data.
3. Uncomplicated fibroids do not cause pelvic pain.
4. There are few facts about chronic pelvic pain of unknown cause, except that most series point out that there is pre-existing psychological morbidity in between 70 and 90% of patients studied.

DISCUSSION POINTS

1. It has been suggested that medroxyprogesterone acetate improves symptoms in cases of chronic pelvic pain due to so-called varicosities of the pelvic veins, and indeed a randomized controlled trial demonstrated this.

Unfortunately, although pelvic venography has demonstrated that varices do exist in the ovarian vessels, there are no adequate control data to illustrate how common this condition might be in the asymptomatic population. Furthermore, the association of psychological problems and pelvic pain is greater than that with pelvic varices.

2. As in premenstrual syndrome, hysterectomy is sometimes resorted to eventually; is this a failure of gynaecologists to evaluate their patients adequately from a psychological perspective?

HORMONE REPLACEMENT TREATMENT (HRT) ★★★★

HISTORY

You may be presented with a woman attending for assessment prior to commencing HRT, though this is more likely to arise in discussion of some other case, such as postmenopausal bleeding, unless the hospital has a dedicated menopause clinic. Nevertheless, in such hospitals, recruiting willing helpers from the menopause clinic is not too difficult.

A history of menopausal symptoms should be sought: in particular you should comment on any vasomotor symptoms, psychological morbidity, psychosexual problems and those related to vaginal dryness, and a history of factors predisposing to osteoporosis, especially a sedentary lifestyle.

You should also make a special point of identifying factors in the history which would make the prescription of HRT controversial, for example a strong family history of breast carcinoma, or genital tract malignancy.

EXAMINATION

The general examination remains important. Significant observations to comment on are blood pressure, signs of hyperlipidaemia (xanthelasma, corneal arcus) and the normality or otherwise of breast examination. Especial comment on vaginal examination should be directed to the degree of oestrogenization of the vulva and vagina.

FACTFILE

1. The postmenopausal population of the UK is increasing dramatically, and the mean life expectancy for women currently approaching the menopause is in the middle 80s.
2. The role of the progesterone component of HRT in inducing breast cancer is unknown, but its use does appear to carry some increased risk.
3. Unopposed oestrogen in women with an intact uterus is associated with an increase in endometrial carcinoma, and should not be used.

DISCUSSION POINTS

1. The role of menopause clinics is an appropriate topic for discussion, since for the majority of women, there is as yet no evidence of benefit from such clinics as opposed to the provision of HRT in a general practice setting. The advantages in terms of obtaining long-term research data are very great indeed. However, the new contracts for general practitioners encourage the establishment of specific menopause clinics in general practice.
2. The effects of oestrogen on lipid profiles pre- and postmenopausally appear contradictory, but evidence suggests that HRT is protective. A history of ischaemic heart disease has been considered a contraindication to hormone replacement, but this is now no longer definitely the case and you may well be asked your opinion on this.

3. Some workers suggest that the effects of topically applied vaginal oestrogens result from their systemic action rather than directly. Vaginally applied creams are very popular for the treatment of atrophic vaginitis, and if they act by being absorbed there are two significant points: the first is that if their action is systemic they might lead to the dangers of endometrial proliferation. The second point is that some women have difficulty applying vaginal creams, and if they act by absorption you might as well give them some ethinyl oestradiol orally.

INFERTILITY ★★★★

DEFINITION

Involuntary failure of a couple to conceive after one 1 year of regular unprotected sexual intercourse.

Primary infertility is defined as above, but there must have been no previous pregnancy to that couple.

Secondary infertility is defined as above except that an earlier pregnancy (including spontaneous or induced abortions) has occurred.

HISTORY

Essentially there are three possible contributory mechanisms in infertility. The first is failure of adequate sperm production or function. Anovulation is the second likely problem, and finally, failure of sperm and egg to meet. The extent of previous investigations is identifiable in history taking.

Investigations into each of these aspects may already have been undertaken, though usually you will be presented with a woman who has been admitted for evaluation, and this is most likely to be laparoscopic hydrotubation. Nevertheless, it is important to establish the likely fertility of the male partner. Another group of patients who are readily recruited are those undergoing reversal of sterilization. The fertility of the male partner is even more important to establish before operation in these women. Thus it is important to establish whether he has been investigated and whether your patient is aware of the result of his semen analysis. In some cases the man will already have fathered children, and this, along with his brief medical history, should be ascertained. Remember a number of drugs – azathioprine, for example – suppress spermatogenesis, and it is a rare coup to obtain such a history if the patient has been admitted for laparoscopy and this is not already known.

A history of irregular painless menses is suggestive of anovulation, though this is by no means invariably the case. The patient may offer a history based on basal body temperature measurements or of treatment with ovulation induction agents (clomiphene may have been prescribed in a woman with oligomenorrhoea without prior laparoscopy).

Failure of egg and sperm to meet may be suggested by a history of coital difficulty and frequency (requires tact), or a history of earlier pelvic inflammatory disease or pelvic surgery.

EXAMINATION

Make specific points of examining the visual fields and checking for goitre, lid lag and galactorrhoea. It is very unlikely that you will be presented with a patient who has thyroid dysfunction or a prolactinoma, but these are important negatives and by mentioning them you illustrate to the examiners that you are familiar with the contribution made by these conditions to anovulatory infertility. These should be part of your clinical practice and really should not take too long.

The pattern of hair distribution is also important, and worthy of comment if obviously abnormal. An apparent increase in body or facial hair distribution, however, relates most strongly to ethnic grouping.

Vaginal examination is usually unremarkable, but make a point of checking that the vaginal tissues are well oestrogenized. Retroversion of the uterus is not a contributor to infertility in the absence of other pelvic disease.

FACTFILE

1. Infertility occurs in 15% of couples. Of these, unexplained infertility occurs in 20–35%.
2. The only proof of ovulation is conception, as the other diagnostic criteria do not exclude defective oocyte release since, in luteinized unruptured follicle syndrome luteinization occurs and progesterone levels rise but the ovum is not actually released.

DISCUSSION POINTS

1. Infertility treatment is no longer considered by some health authorities to be worthy of funding. Who should fund this condition if it is 'not a disease'?
2. Should ovulation induction with gonadotrophins be restricted to specialist units? There is an undoubted association between rates of ovulation induction and multiple pregnancies, as well as ovarian hyperstimulation syndrome.

POSTMENOPAUSAL BLEEDING (PMB) ★★★★

DEFINITION

Bleeding from the genital tract more than 1 year after the last menstrual period (should be considered as caused by genital tract malignancy until proven otherwise).

Common causes
- Atrophic vaginitis ★★★
- Hormone replacement treatment ★★★
- Malignancy of the genital tract ★★

HISTORY

The important point in taking and presenting the history in a case of PMB is to identify risk factors for carcinoma of the genital tract, and endometrial carcinoma in particular. It is particularly important to obtain/exclude a history of hormone replacement treatment or prolonged episodes of anovulation, as in polycystic ovarian syndrome, and when the last cervical smear was taken.

When delivering your history make a point of highlighting positive factors such as a history of diabetes or hypertension or significant negatives such as an absence of a history of hormone replacement treatment.

Because cervical cancer may also present as PMB it is important to avoid becoming too focused on endometrial disease.

EXAMINATION

Often there will be no particularly unusual finding at vaginal examination, but comment if the vagina is atrophic (or obviously well oestrogenized). Remember that the majority of women with cervical carcinoma still present with postmenopausal bleeding, so comment on the normality or otherwise of the cervix. PMB may occasionally be the presenting feature of women with procidentia with an ulcerated cervix, so be prepared to consider and discuss this possibility.

GYNAECOLOGY

1. Only a minority of cases of PMB are actually associated with malignancy. Some workers quote malignancy rates of up to 10% in these women, but this very much reflects referral bias.

2. The vast majority of endometrial carcinomas are adenocarcinoma.

3. Staging of endometrial cancer is surgical.

4. Cervical smears will be abnormal in 68% of women with endometrial carcinoma.

5. The role of progesterone therapy in the management of endometrial carcinoma remains unresolved, as the majority of studies thus far have failed to stratify patients adequately, for example by tumour oestrogen receptor status.

6. Age-specific incidence rates for carcinoma of the cervix show a peak at age 68–70, although there is a small peak at 50 years. The majority of cervical cancers therefore present as post-menopausal bleeding.

7. Ninety-five per cent of cervical cancers are squamous, although the proportion of adenosquamous or adenocarcinomas of the cervix appears to be rising.

8. Staging of cervical cancer is clinical–pathological.

9. Never having had a smear test is now the biggest risk factor for the development of invasive cancer of the cervix in areas where there is a comprehensive cervical cytology service.

10. Hormone replacement therapy is becoming the commonest cause of true PMB. In general practice between 9 and 17% of asymptomatic postmenopausal women receive HRT.

DISCUSSION POINTS

1. At the undergraduate level the focus in discussion will often be on questions of fact, such as the staging of endometrial cancer and what role staging plays in planning management.

2. The value of regular cervical smear tests in reducing cancer of the cervix is a rich source of discussion. Current recommendations are that women be screened every 3 years.

PROLAPSE ★★★★

HISTORY

The history will probably be of a postmenopausal woman complaining of 'something coming down'. There may of course be a history of incontinence, and this will be dealt with separately. The important points in the history relate to risk factors for uterovaginal prolapse, e.g. high parity, obesity, chronic obstructive airways disease. It is said that women who have been involved in occupations associated with physically demanding work are also at high risk.

Prolapse in premenopausal women is not too common, but regardless of the patient's age it is important practically to determine whether she is sexually active. A less enthusiastic approach might be taken in repairing the vagina if the patient is celibate, and it is dangerous to assume that advancing age is invariably associated with reduced sexual activity!

It is important to determine the physical fitness of the patient, as this might influence matters towards a conservative management with ring pessaries. Similarly, the patient's home support is important in planning her care.

EXAMINATION

The general physical examination will allow you to consider the patient's fitness for operation, although if she tells you that she has been admitted for operation it might seem arrogant if you decide she is unfit for anaesthesia. Occasionally an abdominal mass is found in association with prolapse, so make a point of excluding this.

The vaginal examination in this situation allows you to illustrate that you are comfortable in assessing this common problem. Do not rush into asking the patient to strain or cough. In older women the vulva may well be atrophic, and you may have the opportunity to comment on any abnormalities.

Having examined the external genitalia you can then ask the patient to cough. Make a point of asking her to turn her head away from yourself and the examiners at this point. You can then describe the components of the prolapse and its degree. Examination in the left lateral position using a Sim's speculum should not be omitted.

At the conclusion of the examination you can summarize your findings. It may well be that you did not demonstrate a large prolapse, or indeed any prolapse. If so, say so. You may feel that operation is not indicated and, if this is the case, that perhaps physiotherapy may be of benefit. Remember the examiners might be as horrified as you at the idea of someone doing a colporrhaphy on a young woman with no obvious problem!

FACTFILE

1. The failure rate of anterior colporrhaphy is high when the procedure is performed for genuine stress incontinence.
2. Renal failure is a rare consequence of ureteric obstruction due to procidentia.

DISCUSSION POINTS

1. The contribution of cystocoele to stress incontinence in any individual patient is difficult to assess. Abdominal operations such as colposuspension have a role even in moderate cystocoele.
2. Vaginal hysterectomy is more commonly performed in some parts of the UK than others. Why?

URINARY INCONTINENCE ★★★★

DEFINITION

Urinary incontinence is the involuntary loss of urine.

HISTORY

The aim of your history is to determine the probable under-lying pathology. You should by now have met so many women with this problem that you have a well developed system for history taking. However, things you should pay particular attention to are the pattern of fluid intake, as are daytime and nocturnal patterns of micturition. Occasionally you see women with quite amazing patterns of fluid intake who have been admitted for evaluation of incontinence when their addiction to tea would be better treated, so remember and ask. Likewise, particularly in the older woman, determine whether she is receiving treatment with diuretics. You will be used to thinking in terms of genuine stress incontinence and detrusor instability, but remember that physical disability with reduced mobility might un-mask incontinence in a woman who would otherwise have no problem.

Rarely you will be presented with an unusual case of incontinence, such as previous radiotherapy or obstetric or gynaecological trauma resulting in vesicovaginal fistula.

Determine whether the patient has been admitted for physiotherapy and bladder retraining, or for urodynamic assessment. It is more likely, however, that you will meet a patient who has been admitted for definitive surgery for incontinence. There is a big problem here. Anterior colpor-rhaphy is still employed by some gynaecologists for the management of stress incontinence. In the presence of significant cystocoele this may be worthwhile, but in the absence of prolapse is associated with a very poor success rate. Try to determine from the history if there is also a complaint of 'something coming down'.

EXAMINATION

General examination may be rewarding; even in the absence of prolapse there is an association between stress incontinence and smoking, so comment on the respiratory examination.

The vaginal examination will be very important but is only possible when the examiners join you. Exclude prolapse if possible. You must try to demonstrate stress incontinence. A word of warning is that in gross cases the urine can fairly splash out, so stand clear enough to avoid ruining your new suit.

FACTFILE

1. Clinical history is only poorly associated with urodynamic findings.
2. Coughing may induce detrusor contractions and give a false impression of stress incontinence.
3. Urinary retention is rare in the female, but may follow colposuspension, be associated with neurological disorders or, rarely, with a retroverted fibroid or pregnant uterus.

DISCUSSION POINTS

1. Physiotherapy appears to benefit some women with bladder instability, but long-term outcomes are poor. Should inpatient bladder retraining be more widely available?
2. Drug therapy of detrusor instability is poor. The most effective drug, Terodoline, was withdrawn because of a number of cases of sudden death in elderly women.

INTERMENSTRUAL BLEEDING/ABNORMAL SMEAR ★★★

DEFINITION

Intermenstrual bleeding is bleeding from the genital tract between menses in a woman with a regular menstrual cycle and who is not on oral contraception (which might be associated with breakthrough bleeding).

There is a variety of definitions of abnormal cervical smears. A practical smear classification, with appropriate recommendations for action when dealing with 'well women' is given below:

Cytology	Action
Unsatisfactory	Repeat smear soon
Negative	Routine 3-yearly recall
Borderline	Treat infection if present and repeat in 3-months, or 6 months if there is koilocytosis without dyskaryosis
Positive	Colposcopy

Causes

- Cervical polyp ★★★
- Cervical ectopy/cervical intraepithelial neoplasia ★★★
- Cervical carcinoma ★★
- Endometrial carcinoma ★★
- Ovulation bleeding ★
- Oral contraception (properly called breakthrough bleeding, rather than intermenstrual bleeding) ★
- Endometrial polyps ★★

Cervical intraepithelial neoplasia (CIN) ***

The associations of cervical intraepithelial neoplasia are reasonably well established. The specific role of some factors,

GYNAECOLOGY

such as herpes simplex virus (HSV) and human papilloma virus (HPV), is still being elucidated.

Implicated factors:

- HSV infection: This may act as a disease initiator
- HPV infection: Types 16 and 18 have particularly been implicated, but type 18 has also been found in normal tissue
- Multiple sexual partners
- Cigarette smoking
- Young age at first intercourse
- High parity.

HISTORY

Intermenstrual bleeding is a common gynaecological symptom and it is therefore not too difficult to recruit women with this problem for examinations. Alternatively you may be presented with an asymptomatic woman who has been found at a well woman clinic to have a cervical polyp. Cervical screening campaigns are increasing the number of women presenting asymptomatically for evaluation of possible CIN, and these may also be recruited for the purposes of the examination.

The patient may be admitted or attending for colposcopy, conization, or other definitive treatment. In obtaining the history, however, it is important to establish whether post-coital or intermenstrual bleeding has been a problem. Establish aetiological factors, though in the examination it is unwise to upset the patient by asking just how many partners she may have had.

Plans for any further pregnancies might be relevant, as such a desire may influence management of CIN and by obtaining such a history you are illustrating that you are familiar with this.

EXAMINATION

Often no abnormality will be found on general examination. On vaginal examination you may see an ectopy or polyp, but the cervix may appear normal.

FACTFILE

1. Cervical ectopy is the preferred term for erosion, since there is no 'erosive' process, and it is more descriptive of the physiological process.

2. The upper limit of the transformation zone is defined as that area adjoining the lower limit of normal glandular epithelium, and not the upper limit of the squamous epithelium.

3. Colposcopy is mandatory in the management of CIN because it allows directed biopsy with minimal damage to the cervix in the majority of such patients.

DISCUSSION POINTS

1. Cervicography, which involves taking a colposcopic photograph of the cervix, has been suggested as an efficient way of making the expertise of colposcopists available to more women by having technicians photograph the cervix for later examination.

2. You should be familiar with the types of therapy available for treating CIN. These include laser destruction, cold coagulation and knife cone biopsy. Large loop excision of the transformation zone permits excision of the abnormal area using cutting/coagulating diathermy and provides a histological specimen. In this regard it is diagnostic as well as therapeutic, but does not have the drawbacks caused by a formal conization,

which carries the risk of damage to the cervix with later recurrent abortion or premature labour.

3. The value of screening techniques has been well demonstrated, but how frequently smears should be taken for maximum cost/benefit is unknown. You should know the current recommendations.

VAGINAL DISCHARGE ★★★

DEFINITION

There is no standard definition of vaginal discharge, although some textbooks refer to leukorrhoea synonymously with vaginal discharge. Many still reserve this term for a white discharge.

A working definition, however, is the complaint of excessive or unpleasant vaginal secretion which may or may not be accompanied by pruritis and/or unpleasant odour.

HISTORY

The important features are the duration of the symptoms and the exact nature of the problem, i.e. is there an odour or pruritis? A history of previous failed treatment or the use of broad-spectrum antibiotics is important, suggesting the possibility of recurrent candidal vaginitis.

It is unlikely that the patient will be a child, and although foreign bodies are a common cause of vaginal discharge in children they are uncommon in adults. Nevertheless, retained tampons or lost diaphragms still occasionally present and indeed discharge is not uncommon in women with long-standing ring pessaries.

The age of the patient is important, since the aetiology of vaginal discharge is closely linked to age. In this regard it is worth mentioning that a bloodstained discharge in postmenopausal women should be considered as post-menopausal bleeding.

Causes

- Trichomonal infection ★★★
- Candidal infection ★★★
- *Gardnerella vaginalis* infection ★★★
- Chronic cervicitis ★★
- Atrophic vaginitis/endometritis ★★
- Foreign body ★
- Herpes vulvovaginitis ★
- Gonorrhoea ★
- Vaginal adenosis ★

EXAMINATION

Your general examination is aimed at excluding systemic disease, and you should make a point of excluding anaemia and the possibility of diabetes should, if possible, be further investigated by urinalysis. Often in gynaecology no urine specimen may be available, so mention if this is the case. In presenting your history it may be worth commenting that your examination would normally include this investigation.

During the vaginal examination you should specifically identify whether there is any evidence of previous Bartholinitis (you should always palpate for Bartholin's glands but, as you do in the driving test when you exaggerate looking in the mirror, this is one situation when you might emphasize this more).

DISCUSSION POINTS

1. Contact tracing is commonplace within genitourinary medicine, but gynaecologists are awful at this; how might this be achieved in current practice?

2. A proportion of women complain of vaginal discharge when there is no obvious evidence of infection. How should these women be treated? The usual explanation given to the patient is that her discharge is 'physiological'.

3. Should all women undergoing termination of pregnancy be screened for vaginal infection?

VULVAL MASS/PRURITIS VULVAE ★★★

HISTORY

The majority of women who complain of vulval problems will have either a Bartholin's cyst or pruritis. The causes of pruritis have been covered to some extent by the section on vaginal discharge. The other causes usually relate to the vulval epithelial disorders. The history in these cases is usually one of vulval itch in postmenopausal women, though it is also important to exclude – if possible during history taking – other dermatological diseases, including contact dermatitis from the use of an inappropriate deodorant or biological washing powder for example.

Very rarely a psychiatric history might suggest the possibility of a traumatic self-induced dermatitis.

EXAMINATION

General examination should identify systemic disorders such as anaemia.

Care should be taken during the vulval examination to comment on any abnormality in pigmentation.

Any obvious mass should be described appropriately, and it is also important to make a point of examining the inguinal lymph nodes, although this might already have formed part of the general physical examination.

Examine Bartholin's glands and, since the patient is likely to be older, ask her to cough or strain to elicit any signs of uterovaginal prolapse.

FACTFILE

1. The role of pelvic lymphadenectomy for vulval carcinoma is now thought to have been too radical and does not improve long-term prognosis.
2. Human papilloma virus genomes have been identified in vulval intraepithelial neoplasia, and the increasing prevalence of this virus may increase the incidence of vulval malignancy.

DISCUSSION POINTS

1. Bartholin's cysts may be seen in clinical examinations, though they are unlikely to remain as the main topic of discussion. Other vulval lesions are relatively uncommon, but discussion is likely to focus on vulval carcinoma. (Since this carcinoma contributes only 4% to the overall incidence of gynaecological malignancy it is unlikely that you would meet this in the clinical exam. Nevertheless, you are very reasonably expected to recognize a clinically obvious case.) Other, rarer, vulval masses will include vulval fibromas, chancroid and tuberculosis.

2. Pruritis vulvae and its diagnosis and management is probably one of the more disheartening cases to be presented with. This is in part related to the fact that the experts (e.g. the International Society for the Study of Vulval Disease) seem to change the classification of vulval disease just when the average gynaecologist thinks they have mastered the previous one. The important point here is that the correct classification includes the term 'vulval epithelial disorders', but many gynaecologists persist in using the term 'vulval dystrophy'. You should have a clear idea of the descriptive classification system you will use, which should be the one in use in your medical school.

PELVIC MASS ★★

You may fortuitously be presented with a woman who knows that she has been admitted for investigation of, or operation on, a pelvic mass. The majority of women in this situation will be able to tell you what she has actually been admitted with in more specific terms. Relatively few women with ovarian cysts are available to help 'electively' with clinical examinations. In the majority of cases masses palpable in the pelvis are fibroid uterus or loaded bowel. Other possibilities are of more obscure masses, such as pelvic kidney, which occurs fortuitously in the exam. Beware also the full bladder. The list below is certainly not in any way exhaustive, but includes most of the masses you might meet in the gynaecological (and perhaps the surgical) exam.

Causes

- Ovarian cyst ★★★
- Fibroid uterus ★★★★
- Loaded bowel ★
- Full bladder ★
- Pelvic kidney ★
- Retroperitoneal tumour ★
- Crohn's disease ★
- Pelvic abscess ★

HISTORY

You will be familiar with the likely differences in history that distinguish ovarian cysts from fibroids. One important note is that postmenopausal bleeding is not a feature of leiomyomata. In terms of the other possible diagnoses, an adequate history should be helpful in the majority of cases. Crohn's disease may be seen in gynaecology but the diagnosis is usually reached at laparotomy, often to the gynaecologist's embarrassment.

EXAMINATION

In general the features of a pelvic mass should be described in the same way as any other lump, i.e. site, size, shape, consistency, tenderness, bruits, percussion findings etc. The peculiarities of 'gynaecological' lumps include whether they are associated with fluid collections: for example, if presented with an ovarian cyst the possibility of both ascites and pleural effusion should be considered. In terms of small print, if you find an ovarian mass which is associated with a pleural effusion you might mention Meig's syndrome, but this should not be suggested as a likely first diagnosis. Small-print stuff should be kept until last, and only be introduced if you are confident that you can discuss it.

FACTFILE

1. The incidence of ovarian cancer is increasing, but there is no evidence that a greater proportion of cases are being diagnosed earlier. The aetiology is still being established, although certain factors are associated with the disease: a strong family history is important and there appear to be certain oncogenes identified with ovarian neoplasia. Oral contraception may have a beneficial prophylactic effect.

2. Staging is important for all malignancies, but this is particularly the case with ovarian disease as newly developed chemotherapeutic regimens must be compared on a like stage basis with current therapy.

3. Debulking surgery is the only approach that offers cure, and by its nature means that no malignant masses of greater than 1.5 cm in diameter have been left behind at laparotomy.

4. Fibroids are the most common benign tumours in women and have a significant ethnic distribution, being much commoner in black women than other groups.

DISCUSSION POINTS

1. Screening for ovarian cancer. The observation that ovarian cancer usually presents as stage 3 or 4 disease has fostered interest in early diagnosis by the application of population screening. This includes detection by routine pelvic examination and by pelvic ultrasonography coupled with biochemical screening for CA125. The

success of these strategies remains to be determined, but it is likely that many women with benign disease will be identified and may undergo unnecessary laparotomy. This 'trade-off' has to be compared with the potential benefits of early diagnosis. The United States National Institutes of Health recently concluded that screening for ovarian cancer may cause more harm than good. In a cost–benefit analysis they concluded that even if currently available screening tests were ideal and treatment effective, each life saved would cost $1,000 000.

2. The staging of ovarian cancer can often be a fruitful starting point for discussions on further treatment.

3. The degenerations fibroids are likely to undergo are relatively obvious topics for discussion. The benign degenerations are hyaline, cystic, calcific, fatty and red degeneration. Leiomyosarcomata may occur as malignant change in a pre-existing fibroid or as a primary phenomenon. The true incidence of malignant change is unknown, but is certainly, less than 0.5%.

4. Recent evidence suggests that the prognosis for ovarian cancer stage for stage is better in women treated in teaching hospitals. Why might this be?

RECURRENT ABORTION ★★

DEFINITION

Recurrent abortion is the occurrence of three or more consecutive spontaneous abortions.

HISTORY

It is particularly important to establish the obstetric history in some detail. Depending on the interests and orientation of the clinician, some gynaecologists consider recurrent abortion as virtually synonymous with cervical incompetence. There are two main problems with this: the first is that there is no diagnostic test for cervical incompetence, and secondly, there is no proven uniformly effective treatment.

A candidate of quality will be readily capable of taking a history in cases of recurrent abortion, but for a poorly prepared individual this kind of case can be disastrous, so prepare thoroughly.

The length of gestation at the time of the abortion is important, as is the nature of the abortion process, e.g. classically, abortion due to cervical incompetence is associated with a painless presentation following rupture of the membranes and abortion promptly thereafter. It is surprising the number of women thought to have cervical incompetence whose histories include painful vaginal bleeding.

It is important in second-trimester losses to consider the pathological process as being more like the processes of labour, rather than first-trimester loss.

Nevertheless, more attention is now being paid to the genetics and immunology of recurrent abortion. In theory, consanguinity might be expected to increase the risk of miscarriage resulting from immune causes. Consanguinous relationships are also at high risk of expressing autosomal recessive disorders, and this is particularly the case in immigrant communities.

Causes

- Idiopathic ★★★★
- Cervical incompetence ★★★
- Lupus inhibitor/antiphospholipid syndrome ★★
- Balanced translocations in parents ★★
- Hypothyroidism ★
- Uterine abnormalities (Mullerian system) ★

EXAMINATION

A general physical examination should be performed to exclude any general medical disorder, including thyroid disorders. Vaginal examination will only rarely demonstrate any abnormality.

Rarely you will find an abnormality of the vagina or cervix suggesting a uterine anomaly.

FACTFILE

1. Of all pregnancies, 0.4% will be third consecutive spontaneous abortions.
2. The success rate in terms of 'take-home baby rates' for women with recurrent abortion is 68%.
3. There is no proven diagnostic test for cervical incompetence.

DISCUSSION POINTS

1. Antiphospholipid syndrome is being increasingly recognized as a cause of first- and second-trimester spontaneous abortion. Treatment with aspirin and low molecular weight heparins may reduce the loss rate. You could be asked how this might work.
2. Generally, the psychological aspects of the management of pregnancy loss are badly managed. You might be asked how this could be improved.

OBSTETRICS

HISTORY AND EXAMINATION IN OBSTETRICS

PRESENTING THE OBSTETRIC CASE

Candidates often have difficulty presenting the obstetrical history, since in many cases there is no 'presenting complaint'. You should know how to take the past obstetric history in detail. This includes specifics about when previous pregnancies ended, how they ended, e.g. miscarriage, term delivery etc. The mode of delivery and any complications should be specifically enquired about. You may be presented with a patient with a specific problem in pregnancy and who has been admitted. It is important not to concentrate on this alone and miss out previous pregnancies etc.

Beware one small thing: women who have an antepartum haemorrhage may also have pre-eclampsia, so your approach must take this into account. When presented with such a case it is wise to work out how you might deal with each problem individually and then how you might deal with them in combination. One style for presenting your case is outlined below, with some of the relevant comments. In the obstetric case it is useful to start by stating the patient's name, age, parity and gestation, and the problem. Thus you might say, 'I'd like to introduce Mrs Amanda Jones, who is a 24-year-old para 2 + 0 at 32 weeks' gestation who presented with an antepartum haemorrhage'. People have different opinions on which aspect of the history to present next, and to some extent you can direct things as you wish if you continue smoothly. Since it seems useful to review the current pregnancy some like to hear the menstrual history at this stage, so you might continue thus: 'The first day of Mrs Jones' last normal menstrual period was the 21st of July 199X. She has a 28-day cycle and she had not recently used hormonal contraception'. Clearly such a sentence must be modified appropriately, but by mentioning the menstrual history you have effortlessly illustrated that you are aware of the important elements. You may mention if the gestational age was obtained from the patient based on an ultrasound examination, and if there was a discrepancy from menstrual dates. An explanation for any discrepancy should be given, since this will avoid an almost inevitable question from the examiners. Gestational age and its calculation is so fundamental that some examiners will dwell considerably on this. If you fumble on presenting such a basic part of the history they may pounce and ask all about Naegele and his rule. You may outline the remainder of the history of the current pregnancy. When you reach the current admission try to include in your history relevant features: for example, if presenting Mrs Jones' case and you are describing bleeding, mention whether it was painful or painless, and an approximation of the volume. Some questions are terribly obvious and it seems a pity to waste your time and that of the examiners by leaving them to ask 'Was the bleeding associated with pain?'

The examiners may choose to interrupt your presentation of either the history or findings on physical examination. You should be able to adjust so that if they ask you to go on to discuss relevant positive aspects you do this efficiently. This does not excuse you from taking a detailed history: some people will focus heavily on the social aspects of a case, and you will be expected to take a comprehensive history even if you do not have to present it. Similarly, when presenting your physical examination you must present the findings on general examination. It is not sufficient to say 'The heart was normal'. You must present as detailed a cardiovascular examination as might be expected of a candidate in the final MB examination in general medicine. In all likelihood you will be more familiar with the working end of a stethoscope than your examiners. Although the examiners may wish you to focus, for example, on the abdominal findings, they will tell you if this is the case. Equally they may wish you to give the results of a full general examination.

If you have omitted something, for example ophthalmoscopy, then say so. If you say you examined the eyes and they discover you did not (the batteries are flat in the ophthalmoscope) then you deserve to fail for misleading the examiners. It is certainly permissible to say that although you might have wished, time did not permit adequate examination of the eyes.

Similarly the results of urinalysis should be given. 'The nurse did not tell me' is not a good answer.

You will be asked to examine the abdomen for the benefit of the examiners. It is important that you position the patient properly. Make a point of asking her if she is quite comfortable and to tell you if she feels dizzy or nauseated. From these questions the examiners will see that not only are you concerned about your patient's wellbeing, you are also aware of the dangers of supine hypotension syndrome. In this case it is not so much that you are creating a good impression but are not giving a bad one.

It should be impossible to go through your undergraduate training without having to demonstrate your technique of palpation in obstetrics, but do practise this and let someone experienced tutor you before the examination. The rule here is to have an efficient system that will stay with you regardless of the degree of stress you are under. Too many candidates in clinical examinations appear to be touching the abdomen randomly without a systematic approach. Once you have completed your examination you should be able to stop when the relevant information has been obtained. Some people 'poke around' until the examiner interrupts. This does not give a good impression. (In some parts of the world you will find that the style of palpation of the pregnant abdomen is formalized in what are called the Leopold manoeuvres. These consist of answering four questions: What is at the fundus? Where is the fetal back? What is the presenting part? and What is the attitude of the fetus?

You will be invited to present your findings, and a systematic approach is required. A possible outline, adjustable to different situations, is given below:

'On examination, the abdomen is distended consistent with pregnancy. There are no scars but striae gravidarum and a linea nigra are seen. (Examiners sometimes complain about candidates commenting on such obvious things, but others moan a lot more if you omit them.) The size and shape of the uterus, including the symphysis–fundal height of X centimetres, is consistent/not consistent with the gestational age determined from the first day of the last normal menstrual period. There is a single fetus in a longitudinal lie with a cephalic presentation. The back is to the maternal right and the liquor volume is average. The fetal heart rate is X beats per minute.' This is a comprehensive system for presentation and there are few things it cannot cope with. Additional observations might be commented on. For example, if the abdomen is large for dates it is worth commenting if a fluid thrill is present and on the abdominal girth. Remember that at 40 weeks the girth is usually around 40 inches (100 cm). Suitable alterations need to be made for twins, suspected intrauterine growth restriction etc. Of course you may meet an examiner who does not believe in measuring fundal height in centimetres, or in listening to the fetal heart. Perhaps you do not believe in these things either, but you should be able to justify your decision. (Think for a moment about why you listen to the fetal heart. Is there any point to it, and if so, what?)

A minor point about your statement about the size of the uterus being consistent with dates deserves mention. Some people use the term 'equal to so many weeks'. It is not possible to determine gestational age on palpation late in pregnancy. If you base your estimate of gestational age on palpation you will never identify a small-for-dates fetus or a macrosomic fetus. Consequently this phrase is sloppy, despite being in common usage.

Try to leave some time to go through your case before the examiners arrive. It seems a pity that some candidates present a case of pre-eclampsia very well and then, when the examiners ask for a definition of this condition, act as if this is one of the questions they had never considered being asked. The other thing of note is that if you are mentally preparing a list of answers to an anticipated question, for example 'What are the causes of hypertension identified for the first time during pregnancy?', you should start with the most common. Do not lead off with small print. In other words, if you start off with systemic lupus erythematosus as a cause you will both upset the examiners and provoke them into asking you all you know about the dermatological manifestations of SLE in pregnancy.

THE CASES

MULTIPLE PREGNANCY ★★★★★

HISTORY

The vast majority of women with a multiple pregnancy are aware of the fact from early diagnosis by ultrasound. You may be presented with an asymptomatic woman, or alternatively someone admitted with a complication of pregnancy.

The basics of history taking should focus on the relevant facts, i.e. if the presentation is as a result of admission with antepartum haemorrhage then focus initially on this. If the patient is asymptomatic then you may turn early to the issue of the diagnosis of the twin pregnancy.

Multiple pregnancy offers the opportunity to show off the wealth of experience you have acquired in history taking, e.g. women with multiple pregnancies are virtually never entirely asymptomatic, and problems such as heartburn, lethargy, frequency and varicose veins are definitely worthy of comment, but be careful not to overemphasize these.

Increasingly interest focuses on whether ovulation was induced, and this is particularly the case in women with triplets and other higher-order pregnancies.

A family history of twinning is often asked about, but the history on the paternal side is of very limited significance, and on the maternal side it is only a history of dizygotic multiple pregnancy that is associated with an increased risk of having twins.

EXAMINATION

The general examination should be thorough and, since anaemia is one of the commonest complications of multiple pregnancy, the identification of the relevant clinical signs is important. Remember simple things like checking for varicosities. Do not focus on the question of 'twins' alone. Remember that pre-eclampsia is common in multiple pregnancy, so do not omit looking for the signs of this. Many people will make a point of focusing on the abdominal palpation, and will sometimes try to fit the clinical signs to the knowledge that they already have that the case is, for example, twins. The first sign should be that the uterus is large for dates. The often-quoted ways of diagnosing twin pregnancy, i.e. of palpating three fetal poles and of two observers hearing a difference in heart rate, are worthy of some attention: in clinical practice polyhydramnios, a complication of monozygotic twinning, will obviously prevent you from identifying three poles, but in fact even with uncomplicated twin pregnancy this can be enormously difficult.

Although some examiners say that ultrasound has taken the fun out of diagnosing twins and has led to a reduction in diagnostic skills, they often forget that before the widespread use of ultrasound, 50% of twins were unidentified until labour.

If the uterus is not large for dates then consider the possibility of intrauterine growth restriction, although this can not readily be diagnosed clinically. Do not be afraid to say that the uterus is not as large as you might expect to find, since you can highlight the difficulties of diagnosing IUGR in twin pregnancy.

Finally, if the uterus feels 'irritable' during palpation this is also worthy of comment. By your examination thus far you have sought signs of or demonstrated that you are aware of the most common perinatal problems in multiple pregnancy.

1. The incidence of twin pregnancy, quoted as 1 per 80 pregnancies, is increasing, largely as a result of assisted conception techniques such as ovulation induction, GIFT and IVF.
2. Dichorionicity is not synonymous with dizygosity.
3. The perinatal mortality rate in twin pregnancy is increased between 6 and 10 times that of singletons, and is largely due to the higher rates of fetal abnormality and premature delivery.

DISCUSSION POINTS

1. Almost all of the complications of pregnancy, are commoner in multiple pregnancy, so examiners can use this as a springboard to discuss anything from haematinic deficiency to preterm labour. Consequently, you can reasonably expect to be asked anything at all about obstetrics!
2. Some obstetricians will ask about the practical obstetrical aspects of multiple pregnancy, and will ask about the problems of delivery of the second twin and the methods of identifying fetal lie and position.

NORMAL PREGNANCY ★★★★★

Although there are definitions of normal labour there are no widely accepted definitions of normal pregnancy, although most obstetricians know what they think they mean by the term. Those who are given the task of organizing cases for clinical examinations frequently find difficulty in recruiting large numbers of hypertensive diabetics in renal failure at 36 weeks' gestation. This means that there is a distinct possibility of being presented with a woman who appears to be going through an uncomplicated pregnancy. There are a number of reasons why such a woman might be helping with the exam. The first is that she is there not because of a current problem but because of some problem in a previous pregnancy, for example previous caesarean section; secondly she may actually have a problem but neither you nor she is aware of it. An example of this might be the woman who has mild anaemia but nobody has told her, and the time that you find out is when the examiner says something like 'and what if I told you that Mrs Jones's haemoglobin is 8.9 g%?' The last reason might be that the senior registrar organizing the exam has run out of pre-eclamptics, and the placenta praevia she arranged for you started bleeding 20 minutes ago and is currently being delivered.

Your history taking must be even more comprehensive in these circumstances, since the examiners can choose virtually any topic for discussion, and if they are given the information that the patient is 'normal' then they will have high expectations of the quality of the history.

EXAMINATION

As with the history taking your examination should be fairly comprehensive, but do not forget that you may find a problem which neither the organizers nor the examiners are aware of. Examples might be that you consider the uterus to be small for dates, or that there is a breech presentation. In other words there may be a problem which you are the first to identify, and this is a wonderful opportunity if you grasp it.

DISCUSSION POINTS

1. The expectation by parents that their children will be entirely normal is being made increasingly likely by

the increasingly widespread use of prenatal diagnosis techniques. You should be aware of the recommendations of the 23rd study group of the RCOG, among which is the statement that routine anomaly scanning should be performed at 18–20 weeks, and preferably be preceded by a dating scan in early pregnancy.

2. You should be familiar with the routine pattern of antenatal care in your area. The contribution of general practitioners to antenatal and intrapartum care has recently attracted considerable attention and would be worthy of mention.

POST-DATES PREGNANCY ★★★★★

DEFINITION

Pregnancy proceeding to 42 completed weeks gestation.

HISTORY

This comes back to the importance of accurate dating, therefore the menstrual history is crucial and the comments about dating mentioned in the section on the small-for-dates pregnancy are equally valid. If the patient is aware of her dates by early ultrasound then these may be used with justification. Accurate dating in early pregnancy reduces the population incidence of post-dates pregnancy. One of the worst situations to be presented with is a late booker who is 'past dates', so ensure that even in such a case you obtain as clear an idea of dates as possible.

Clinicians' anxieties about adequate functioning of the placenta mean that your history should try to identify fetal condition by, for example, enquiring about fetal activity.

EXAMINATION

There are no specific features to seek in these cases except to note your clinical impression of liquor volume and fetal size. Clinical identification of macrosomia can be difficult, especially in the obese, who comprise a high-risk group for large fetuses.

FACTFILE

1. Perinatal mortality increases twofold after 42 weeks.
2. The caesarean section rate is also increased twofold after 42 weeks.
3. Meconium staining occurs in 30% of pregnancies beyond 42 weeks.

DISCUSSION POINT

The methods available for inducing labour should be familiar to you, and may well be asked about in discussing post-dates pregnancy.

PRE-ECLAMPSIA ★★★★★

DEFINITION

Pre-eclampsia is a condition of unknown aetiology occurring usually in the second half of pregnancy, usually in primigravidas, and characterized by hypertension, proteinuria and oedema.

It is astonishing how a simple question such as 'What is pre-eclampsia?' can upset candidates. Perhaps they are assuming that the examiner wishes to be informed of some of the classifications of hypertension in pregnancy, but let him ask this directly.

Similarly some candidates may feel they have to define further every part of the definition, by saying that hypertension is defined as an increase of 30 mmHg in systolic readings over first-trimester systolic readings or 15 mmHg over first-trimester diastolic recordings, or arbitrarily as a blood pressure of 140/90 mmHg.

Alternatively some candidates are too suspicious and will confuse themselves by wondering why the examiner did not ask what pregnancy-induced hypertension is. Indeed, are pregnancy-induced hypertension and pre-eclampsia different conditions? Do not be too clever. By all means, if you know 24 classifications for hypertension occurring during pregnancy then offer them, if asked, but some examiners will become a shade bothered if you present a case of a woman with 4 g of proteinuria and a blood pressure of 200/105 mmHg and you quibble about which variant of pregnancy-induced hypertension this might be. If it is common or garden pre-eclampsia then you will be expected to appreciate that.

HISTORY

The important points in the history usually relate to risk factors for pre-eclampsia, and you should exclude points in the history suggestive of possible secondary causes. Previous hypertension on the oral contraceptive pill is worthy of comment. Family history is also important, given the high incidence of pre-eclampsia in first-degree relatives of women with the condition.

The history of previous pregnancies is important, since the recurrence risk for previous severe pre-eclampsia is between 18 and 25%, far higher even than most obstetricians consider.

EXAMINATION

Almost certainly you will find no significant abnormality on general examination, with the exception perhaps of elevated blood pressure and some evidence of oedema. However, on general examination it is worth identifying secondary signs of hypertension, and in particular it is worth examining the optic fundi.

Almost certainly the findings will be unremarkable, but such observations are significant negatives and illustrate for the examiners the thoroughness of your approach. An adequate neurological examination is similarly important and you should take pains to exclude an obvious increase in reflexes, although it is unlikely that you will be presented with such a case. Despite the fact that pretibial oedema is a virtually useless sign in obstetrics, many examiners will insist on you demonstrating your ability to elicit it. There are three sites for testing for oedema around the foot (the dorsum of the foot, behind the medial malleolus and pretibially) and you should be able to demonstrate these. More clinically useful is the observation of conjunctival oedema, and if you find this it is worth demonstrating it for the benefit of the examiners.

A thorough examination should not take so much time that you are not able to check the blood pressure and perform a urinalysis. Do not forget the fetal side of the condition, and think carefully about whether the baby is appropriately grown or not.

Remember that in some women with essential hypertension (not pre-eclamptics) the fetus is actually well grown, and these women are said to have made good physiological adjustment to their pregnancies.

1. The incidence of pre-eclampsia varies dramatically depending on the diagnostic criteria used. If one simply uses the definition of a blood pressure of 140/90 mmHg at some time in the second half of pregnancy, then the diagnosis will be made in 25% of primigravidas. If stricter criteria are met, including significant proteinuria, then the incidence is between 5 and 8%.

2. There is substantial evidence to support a genetic disposition to pre-eclampsia, since it is commoner among the sisters, daughters and mothers of women with the disease, though not among matched controls.

3. The endocrine and vascular alterations characterizing pre-eclampsia are identifiable in the second trimester and precede the clinical signs.

4. The common causes of maternal death in pre-eclampsia are cerebrovascular accident and haemorrhage.

5. The role of antihypertensive medication in severe pre-eclampsia is well established, but randomized controlled trials of hypotensive treatment in mild/moderate pre-eclampsia provide equivocal evidence at best.

DISCUSSION POINTS

1. The classification of hypertension in pregnancy is a topic about which some obstetricians can become quite excited. It is wise to have a clear idea of what is meant by the terms pre-eclampsia, pregnancy-induced hypertension and superimposed pre-eclampsia.

2. The issue of bed rest is often brought up in discussion of these cases. The actual bed rest is of dubious value, but admission to hospital does allow frequent measurement of blood pressure and urinalysis.

PREVIOUS CAESAREAN SECTION ★★★★★

DEFINITIONS

The definitions which might be used in this context are those of primary elective caesarean section and emergency caesarean section. The former describes a section undertaken before labour in a woman who has not previously undergone section. Emergency section is a term usually used to describe abdominal delivery undertaken during labour and which may or may not have been preceded by a previous caesarean section. This is not always a useful definition, since a section undertaken at 29 weeks for fulminant pre-eclampsia has clearly been performed in response to an 'emergency', but is often not classified as such.

HISTORY

This is fundamentally an extension of your conventional obstetric history. However, in the context of a previous emergency caesarean section the duration of the labour and the indication for section assume even greater importance. The patient may be able to tell you whether there was a malposition. She should be able to discuss whether she is to be electively 'sectioned' in the current pregnancy. This decision may have been based on the findings at postnatal radiological pelvimetry.

Unfortunately, many women remain seemingly poorly informed about either the plans for their future management or the reasons for their previous management.

Almost all obstetric proformas include a section to be completed on previous pelvic injury. This is very rare, but make a point of excluding this or, in patients in high-risk groups such as certain ethnic communities, enquire about rickets.

Previous elective section is most likely to have been performed for a breech presentation, but other factors should be explored.

EXAMINATION

The general examination may well be totally unremarkable but take special note of the patient's height. Do not take her word for it: it is amazing the number of people who are unsure how tall they are. If possible, and if it seems particularly relevant, you might even ask if the height can be checked, as some women will claim to be quite different from the height recorded in the notes the examiners will have access to.

Obviously on abdominal palpation there will be a scar, but it is remarkably easy to report your findings and forget to mention it, particularly if a Pfannenstiel incision has been used. Beware commenting on whether a caesarean section was 'classic' or not. Midline incisions used to be commonly used for all abdominal deliveries, and consequently most such incisions were used for lower-segment operations as well as classic operations. Some obstetricians feel they can deliver a very preterm baby by classic section through a Pfannenstiel. Happily this is uncommon, but it highlights the necessity for accurate history taking, and if there is doubt in your history then you should mention to the examiners that you would contact the centre where the previous delivery occurred if you did not have access to the relevant data. Do not be confused about this: just be aware that the abdominal incision does not necessarily indicate the nature of the uterine incision.

FACTFILE

1. The caesarean section rate in the UK is rising and the major contributing factors are dystocia (failure to progress), presumed fetal distress (without fetal blood sampling) and previous caesarean section. 'Failure to progress' is not a diagnosis and most cases of caesarean section will result from poorly managed malposition or dysfunctional labour in a primigravida.

2. There is only one commonly used classification of pelvic shape, and describes the pelvis as android, anthropoid, platellypoid or gynaecoid based upon radiological pelvimetry. This classification has never been tested prospectively in current practice. There is no good evidence that radiological pelvimetry, either post caesarean section or intra-partum is of any value whatsoever in the management of subsequent pregnancies.

3. Uterine rupture occurs in 1.5% of previous caesarean sections and is approximately 10 times commoner following classic section compared with the lower segment operation.

DISCUSSION POINTS

1. The selected method of delivery in a woman with a previous section provides the usual topic for discussion and you should be prepared to talk about what factors would influence you toward or away from vaginal delivery.

2. The high section rate and methods of reducing this are fair topics which indicate the clinical exposure of the candidate.

3. General practitioner units could safely be involved in the management of women with a previous section. Discuss.

OBSTETRICS

SMALL FOR DATES (SFD) ★★★★★

DEFINITION

A fetus which is below an arbitrary centile value of weight for gestational age. Some centres use the 10th centile, but an increasing number use the fifth centile and some the third. The third centile identifies a subset which more accurately pinpoints fetuses likely to be genuinely growth restricted *in utero* as well as SFD. It is worth making a small point here: the term growth 'restriction' is increasingly being used in place of the more usual growth 'retardation'. 'Restriction' should be the preferred term, not only because it more actually describes the pathophysiology but also because its use is preferable to parents, for whom the term retardation may have other alarming associations.

It is important to distinguish clearly between intrauterine growth restriction (IUGR) and being SFD. Failure of a fetus to meet its genetically determined growth velocity is the prime feature of IUGR, but not one which can be recognized clinically.

Cases may be recognized by observing a reduction in fetal growth velocity as evidenced by serial ultrasound measurements, but in clinical practice as well as the clinical examination you are more likely to be presented with a clinically SFD fetus. (It is important to appreciate that from the definition of IUGR a fetus need not be SFD to be suffering growth restriction, but this is a concept that many clinicians are uncomfortable with.)

Causes of SFD

- Wrong dates ★★★
- IUGR ★★★★★
- Constitutional ★★★★★
- Ethnic ★★★
- Fetal anomaly ★★

- Maternal smoking ★★★★
- Drug abuse ★★
- Fetal infection ★
- Pre-eclampsia ★★★★
- Previous SFD ★★★★★

HISTORY

Many of the women who are thought to be SFD will be recruited to the examination either while they are inpatients admitted for evaluation or attending a day unit for fetal assessment. Consequently, most will be aware that there may be a problem with fetal growth or wellbeing.

It is important not to be side-tracked by the immediate issue of evaluating the fetus: the important point is to establish whether the fetus is actually SFD. The first issue, therefore, is whether the dates are accurate. Some examiners will focus very heavily indeed on menstrual data. You must establish the gestational age from dates as reliably as possible, and if there is doubt about the dates any additional information is essential. Clearly many women will be aware of the gestational age derived from an ultrasound examination. You should be aware of the likely accuracy of ultrasound estimation of gestational age, since in women who book late in the second trimester ultrasound is not much more help in dating than a history of when quickening was noted.

The past obstetric history is one of the most important parts of the history, since the single largest risk factor for the delivery of a SFD fetus is a previous event. Birth order is also important, and therefore a clinically SFD fetus in a women who has previously delivered well grown fetuses raises anxiety about fetal normality. Social history is very important insofar as it is known that smoking and drug abuse are associated with SFD fetuses.

The history of the pregnancy from the first trimester may be helpful, since other factors are associated with SFD cases and may have been forgotten by the patient, e.g. elevated maternal serum alpha-fetoprotein (AFP) in mid-trimester. If the patient did have such a finding then she will probably have undergone detailed sonography, or may already have had a structural survey. The exclusion of major fetal anomaly may well have been achieved already, although it is important to remember that there is no established ultrasound technique for excluding trisomies when there is no accompanying structural anomaly.

EXAMINATION

General examination is designed to identify potential causes of SFD and possibly IUGR. Comment on physical evidence suggesting heavy smoking or evidence of chronic disease.

The main issue by the time you come to examine the abdomen will be whether fetal size is consistent with the gestational age you have arrived at. You must ask yourself if the uterus really is SFD. The clinical signs associated with IUGR are that the uterus is SFD, the fetus feels flexed, the liquor volume feels reduced and the fetal parts are more readily felt.

FACTFILE

1. Recognition of the SFD fetus is notoriously difficult, and this might lead some people to a sense of nihilism since only 50% of SFD fetuses are actually identified as such. This relatively poor sensitivity in detection is matched by the fact that, of every three fetuses suspected of being SFD, only one actually is.

DISCUSSION POINTS

The most frequent problems in the management of suspected SFD cases are the resolution of the accuracy of gestational age assessment, the question of when to deliver, and how to evaluate fetal wellbeing before this. Most evaluation is based on biophysical assessment, particularly cardiotocography.

Biophysical profile screening, introduced as an intra-uterine version of the Apgar score, evaluates five parameters of fetal wellbeing. These are cardiotocography, liquor volume, the presence of fetal body movements, fetal breathing movements and fetal tone. If you are asked to outline the management of a case of suspected SFD fetus, never use phrases like 'I would monitor fetal wellbeing'. The word 'monitor' should be avoided and replaced with specifics. In other words, if you want to arrange daily cardiotocography and twice-weekly biophysical profiles, then say so.

ANTEPARTUM HAEMORRHAGE (APH) ★★★★

DEFINITION

Bleeding from the genital tract from 24 weeks' gestation to delivery.

Causes

- Placenta praevia ★★★★ A condition wherein the placenta or a part thereof lies in the lower uterine segment (the lower uterine segment is that part of the uterus which lies below the reflection of the uterovesical peritoneum).
- Placental abruption ★★ A condition in which a normally sited placenta separates prematurely from the uterine wall.
- Marginal haemorrhage ★★★
- Cervical polyp/polyp ★★★
- Cervical carcinoma ★
- Spurious causes include haematuria and rectal bleeding ★

HISTORY

When you are presented with a woman who gives a history of vaginal bleeding the important features are: when the bleeding occurred, an estimate of the volume, whether it was associated with abdominal pain and whether it was postcoital.

Repeated episodes of bleeding are a feature of placenta praevia, so be careful when you ask when the bleeding occurred: you may find the patient tells you about the most recent event, and not any earlier episodes. Clinicians' estimates of vaginal bleeding are pretty awful and patients themselves are not particularly good, since to an anxious woman a small volume may look like major haemorrhage. Bleeding which is heavier or lighter than a period is a useful distinction, since the woman at least has a reference point. A history such as 'the bed was soaked' is useful, but most women whose pregnancies get to the stage of helping with examinations will have a history of lighter bleeding, and you might ask if the blood soaked through her underwear or not. These are more useful reference points than asking someone to estimate if the volume lost was equivalent to a cupful etc. Painful bleeding is said to identify abruption rather than placenta praevia, but if a woman is in preterm labour she may complain of painful contractions while bleeding from a low-lying placenta. Tactful enquiry about whether the bleeding was postcoital is worthwhile, and may even be a significant negative.

When taking the history in the examination setting it is understood that further investigations might have been performed; for example, you may reasonably ask the patient whether she is aware of the site of the placenta from a previous ultrasound scan.

It is also worth asking the patient about findings from earlier investigation; in particular, did she have a cervical smear in the recent past, and if so does she know the result?

EXAMINATION

It is important to confirm on general examination that there is no evidence of anaemia or other sign of recent significant blood loss. Hypertension is a more likely finding than being presented with a hypotensive shocked woman!

On abdominal palpation you should try to identify pointers towards or away from a diagnosis of placenta praevia: clearly a transverse lie or very high presenting part are suggestive, but do not forget that your patient may be having recurrent small abruptions and consider that the uterus might be small for dates. In other words, remember that other diagnoses should be considered. The examiners might be fed up hearing about antepartum haemorrhage and be looking for something else to discuss.

It is unlikely that you will meet a woman in the examination with a tense hard abdomen and absent fetal heart, but you should be prepared to discuss the findings you would anticipate in severe abruption.

FACTFILE

1. APH complicates 2–4% of pregnancies.
2. Before the introduction of conservative management of placenta praevia the fetal loss rate was over 80%.
3. Performing a vaginal examination in a woman presenting with APH without either prior (reliable) knowledge of the placental site or outwith an operating theatre with facilities for immediate delivery is punishable by death (of the patient). Do not let an examiner try to talk you into saying that the clinical diagnosis of abruption is so easy that you should go ahead and rupture the membranes in the ordinary delivery room.

DISCUSSION POINTS

1. It is very easy to confuse candidates about the management of placenta praevia, particularly when some talk about EUA (examination under anaesthesia) and EWA (examination without anaesthetic). These confusing terms might indicate that examination is performed under anaesthetic or without anaesthetic respectively, but remember that 'with' and 'without' both begin with W, and the conservative management of placenta praevia is so very well defined that you should be familiar with its principles. The availability of placentography has, of course, changed the approach to the management of APH, but the clinical examination setting tests knowledge of basic principles as much as knowledge of new techniques.

2. One new technique which is currently being advocated for the reliable diagnosis of placenta praevia is transvaginal ultrasound. This contravenes rules about vaginal examination, although the ultrasound probe clearly does not come into contact with the cervix. You may be asked to comment on this.

BREECH PRESENTATION ★★★★

DEFINITION

Breech presentation is pretty much self-explanatory, but you must be able to define the types of breech presentation: flexed breech is a breech presentation with flexion at the knees and hips. Frank breech describes flexion at the hips and extension at the knees. Footling presentation is said to be an incomplete breech presentation, i.e. one or both feet or knee(s) presents.

HISTORY

You may be presented with a patient who is attending to help with the examination purely because of a breech presentation (in which case part of her history will address this specifically), or breech presentation may be incidental to her attendance either to help with the examination or for routine antenatal care. In this case she may not mention the fact of breech presentation (or even be aware of it). As the incidence of breech presentation is closely related to gestational age, the earlier the gestation of any patient you see the greater the chance of finding a breech presentation. Remember that a case of pre-eclampsia may still also be complicated by a breech presentation, but it is worth analysing your management of each of these problems individually before amalgamating your approach for the more complex situation.

The specific features to note if presented with a case of breech presentation are to determine the gestation when the diagnosis was made, the obstetrician's response (e.g. has the patient undergone external cephalic version?), and what investigations relevant to breech presentation have been arranged.

Try to identify or exclude factors leading to breech presentation: high parity, abnormal uterine shape and multiple pregnancy are always mentioned in the textbooks, but in the majority of women there will not be much in the way of specific facts in the history, although previous breech presentation is a risk factor in a subsequent pregnancy.

The undoubted association with fetal anomaly is important, and a history of satisfactory detailed ultrasound examination is reassuring. Placentography may have been performed, and it is worth asking if the patient is aware whether this has been done.

EXAMINATION

One of the more reassuring comments in one of the standard textbooks is that there is no characteristic finding on abdominal palpation. This is reassuring for practising obstetricians, since failure to identify a breech presentation antenatally is not as uncommon as is thought among those who do not visit labour wards very often. Such people miss the opportunity to determine the accuracy or otherwise of their palpation. The point of all this is that if on palpation the diagnosis is not too obvious, it is no crime to say so.

The clinical features of breech presentation need not be rehearsed here except to mention that occasionally in a cephalic presentation the breech will be ballotable in the fundus, and this can be confusing since some think that a ballotable pole in the fundus must be the head.

Secondly, even if you think the fetal head is well down in a cephalic presentation, beware missing a breech presentation, which can feel very similar to a well-engaged head on abdominal palpation. The final thing to say about examination of a presumed breech presentation is that just because a woman is kind enough to agree to help with the examination when she is seen at the antenatal clinic the week before, this does not preclude the possibility of spontaneous version. Consequently, if you are certain she has a cephalic presentation then say so, even if the patient insists that she has a breech presentation and only agreed to help with the exam in order to have an external cephalic version.

1. Breech presentation occurs in 3% of deliveries at term, but is found in 28% of pregnancies at 28 weeks' gestation and 10% at 32 weeks.
2. The uncorrected perinatal mortality rate in vaginal breech deliveries is 25%, but this reflects two main features: the first of these is the problem of fetal anomaly and its association with breech presentation, and the second is the problem of prematurity, since preterm delivery is more likely to be associated with breech presentation.

DISCUSSION POINTS

1. The management of breech presentation provides a rich source of amusement for examiners. The fundamental fact is that there is no correct answer about the ideal mode of delivery for any breech fetus (almost regardless of gestation).
2. The principal areas of controversy relate to the value of external cephalic version and the mode of delivery.
3. The contraindications to version can also provoke interesting discussion. The list usually given is:
   - planned caesarean section
   - previous caesarean section (hysterotomy)
   - multiple pregnancy
   - placenta praevia
   - antepartum haemorrhage
   - fetal abnormality.

LARGE FOR DATES ★★★

Unlike the term 'small for dates' there is no standard definition of large for dates. A functional definition might be that the uterus is large-for-dates if uterine size is greater than might normally be expected for the given gestation.

Macrosomia is the term used to describe a fetus which is above an arbitrary fetal weight. In North American textbooks macrosomia is used to describe fetuses weighing 4 kg or more. In British practice a 4.5 kg cut-off point is more commonly used.

Causes
- Wrong dates ★★★
- Multiple pregnancy ★★★★
- Macrosomic fetus (including diabetic pregnancy) ★★★
- Gravid fibroid uterus ★★
- Polyhydramnios ★★★★

POLYHYDRAMNIOS

This term describes excessive liquor volume. Again there is no standard definition of polyhydramnios, but the term is used widely to describe the situation where the liquor volume is thought to be excessive. Liquor volume varies markedly with gestation, and even within a single gestational age there is a wide variation.

Causes
- Idiopathic ★★★★
- Anencephaly ★★
- Open spina bifida ★
- Gastroschisis ★
- Exomphalos ★
- Oesophageal atresia ★★★
- Duodenal atresia ★★★
- Hydrops fetalis ★

- Pierre Robin syndrome ★
- Monozygotic twin pregnancy ★★
- Diabetes ★★★

HISTORY

The importance of gestational age and its calculation is as relevant here as in the small-for-dates fetus.

The history in cases of polyhydramnios is variable: the patient may be aware that she is thought to be large but be asymptomatic. The history in symptomatic polyhydramnios is usually of a relatively acute increase in uterine size. This might present with the patient actually complaining of a feeling of her skin being stretched, or with marked oesophageal reflux or worsening haemorrhoids or varicose veins.

You should be able to determine from the patient which investigations have already been performed and identify which of the possible causes have probably already been excluded.

EXAMINATION

General examination in cases of polyhydramnios will confirm peripheral oedema and allow you to identify lower limb varices.

On abdominal palpation the important thing is to identify whether the uterus is actually large for dates. The important points are to determine which of the uterine contents are present excessively and, having done so, being logical in your presentation. It is difficult to take seriously a candidate who says that the liquor volume is markedly increased but that the fetal parts are easily felt and the fetal heart readily heard etc.

The fundal height should be measured in centimetres, and traditionally the abdominal girth in inches. Try to elicit a fluid thrill.

DISCUSSION POINTS

1. The differential diagnosis of large for dates is interesting, since the exclusion of the commoner diagnoses covers many areas of obstetrics, from gestational diabetes to screening for neural tube defect.

2. The importance of diagnosing the macrosomic fetus is much less emphasized in British obstetric practice than in American, but the importation of the same attitudes to litigation may result in an increasing focus on this. The background to this is the higher incidence of obstructed labour and of shoulder dystocia. The possible adverse neurological sequelae in severe shoulder dystocia have led to enormous efforts to improve the identification of large babies.

3. Ultrasound estimation of fetal weight is inaccurate in the large fetus. Those who suggest that ultrasound may be used to identify fetuses at risk of shoulder dystocia have not critically assessed the literature. The mean error in estimation is about 8%, but the 95% confidence limits for an estimated weight of 4 kg is approximately 2.9–4.6 kg.

MEDICAL DISORDERS IN PREGNANCY
(excluding diabetes) ★★★

The approach to medical disorders in pregnancy should address two areas, the effect of the disease on the pregnancy, and the effect of the pregnancy on the disease.

The more common disorders you are likely to meet are:

- Epilepsy ★★★★
- Hyperthyroidism ★★
- Asthma ★★★★
- Cardiac disease (usually asymptomatic) ★★
- Essential hypertension ★★★
- Anaemias (including haemoglobinopathies) ★★★

Epilepsy and its interaction with pregnancy exemplifies the value of a logical approach to the resultant problems. The effect of epilepsy on pregnancy is mediated by both the disease and its treatment. Presumed hypoxic episodes during *grand mal* seizures may play some role in the higher incidence of fetal anomalies seen in the infants of epileptics. This higher incidence of fetal abnormality is a feature of the disease, rather than the drugs used in treatment. Nevertheless, it is likely that all drugs used in the management of epilepsy are teratogenic to some extent: sodium valproate and phenytoin are always mentioned in this regard, but even carbamazepine is now recognized as causing some malformations. Sodium valproate has a significant association with neural tube defect.

Pregnancy has a variable effect on the frequency of convulsions, though when this worsens management problems are compounded by the difficulty of monitoring therapeutic levels in pregnancy.

Epilepsy is also the paradigm for prepregnancy rationalization of treatment since reduction in the dosage or number of anticonvulsants will reduce the risk of malformation. In women with idiopathic epilepsy it may be possible to stop therapy in early pregnancy if the patient has been fit-free for 2 or more years.

Essential hypertension merits further mention, since the effect of mild or moderate hypertension in pregnancy is probably not particularly adverse. The value of treating moderate hypertension in pregnancy is not proven. Atenolol, if given from early in the second trimester, is associated with IUGR and fetal death. Methyldopa appears to be safe throughout pregnancy and has the merit of long-term follow-up data. Pre-eclampsia superimposed on essential hypertension is bad news, but there is no evidence that lowering blood pressure in early pregnancy reduces the risk of this developing.

Finally, anaemia is yet another area where some obstetricians will expect you to be able to discuss the physiology of iron and folate metabolism at length.

In cosmopolitan areas there is a distinct possibility of meeting a patient with one of the haemoglobinopathies. This affords you the possibility of showing off your knowledge of the effect of the disease on the pregnancy with particular regard to the role of prenatal diagnosis. If your examiner is not from an area of large immigrant populations then your knowledge of the genetics of the thalassaemias could impress!

Deep venous thrombosis is clinically very important and its exclusion may be relevant in any of your gynaecological or obstetrical cases. Obtain a detailed history of the previous event. A family history may be important: the contribution of deficiencies in antithrombin III, protein C, protein S and the presence of Leiden factor is being increasingly recognized.

EXAMINATION

The important point is to elicit the physical signs pertinent to the underlying medical disorder.

PRETERM PREMATURE RUPTURE OF THE MEMBRANES (PROM) ★★★

DEFINITION

Rupture of the membranes without establishment of labour before 37 weeks' gestation.

NB: There is considerable confusion about the meaning of premature rupture of the membranes. Without the prefix 'preterm' this is used in North America to describe rupture of the membranes before labour is established, regardless of the gestational age.

HISTORY

The history in cases of suspected rupture of the membranes is usually straightforward: the patient complains of leaking fluid vaginally. This may have begun in a gush of fluid or, alternatively, with a continuous leak of small volumes of fluid. The likeliest source of confusion is with urinary incontinence, which is surprisingly (to some) common in pregnancy.

The gestation at which the membranes ruptured and the duration of PROM should be established. You should try to exclude the more serious sequelae of PROM, particularly chorionamnionitis. A history of flu-like illness should therefore be elicited if possible.

Check whether a speculum examination was performed and whether any bacteriological swabs were taken to exclude infection. Similarly, it may be that liquor was collected for measurement of the lecithin/sphingomyelin ratio and the identification of phosphatidyl glycerol. Clearly not all women would be able to tell you what investigations might have been performed, but you may be lucky.

Similarly you might try to elicit a history of whether steroids were administered to accelerate fetal lung maturity. If rupture of the membranes occurs at term and your patient has been recruited to help with the exam, then she will probably be able to tell you whether a plan has been decided upon to induce labour.

EXAMINATION

On general examination you need to exclude signs of infection, particularly tachycardia and pyrexia. The absence of such signs is worthy of comment.

On abdominal examination exclude uterine tenderness and comment on any reduction in liquor which is clinically obvious. Remember that just because you think the liquor volume should be reduced in cases of PROM, this does not mean that it will be clinically apparent. If you think the liquor volume is normal then have the courage to say so, as the examiners will not be impressed if you say there is oligohydramnios when in fact they find the volume to be clinically normal.

FACTFILE

1. The processes leading to rupture of the membranes are incompletely understood, but it is known that the collagen content of amnion reduces towards term.
2. *Escherichia coli, Bacteroides fragilis* infection and the presence of beta-haemolytic streptococci have been found in association with preterm PROM, but their role in causing a breach in the membranes is unknown.

DISCUSSION POINTS

1. You will be expected to be familiar with the policy relating to the use of steroids to accelerate fetal lung maturity.
2. PROM lends itself to discussion on what factors influence the onset of labour.

PREVIOUS POSTPARTUM HAEMORRHAGE (PPH) ★★★

DEFINITION

Primary postpartum haemorrhage is defined as vaginal bleeding of 500 mls or more within 24 hours of delivery. Secondary PPH is not quantified by volume, but is 'excessive' vaginal bleeding more than 24 hours after delivery until 6 weeks postpartum.

Causes

- Atonic uterus ★★★
- Retained placenta/placental part ★★★★
- Trauma, particularly cervical ★★★

HISTORY

If the only abnormality you have detected in the history is of a previous PPH then the likelihood is that the current pregnancy is normal. Alternatively, there is something you have missed but do not panic.

The important parts of the history to determine are: when the bleeding occurred in relation to delivery, whether the patient became 'unwell', whether blood transfusion was required, and finally, whether examination was undertaken in theatre.

FACTFILE

1. PPH is the most common cause of severe hypotension in obstetric practice.
2. Prolonged labour, multiple pregnancy and polyhydramnios are all associated with PPH, but the commonest cause, since it is invariably associated with loss of more than 500 ml, is caesarean section. Any obstetrician who gives an estimated blood loss of less than 500 ml at caesarean section is either conceited or amazingly optimistic.

DISCUSSION POINTS

1. The normal management of the third stage of labour is a favourite question for students. Similarly, knowledge of the pharmacology of ergometrine and oxytocin is essential, as is how a case of primary PPH should be managed.

2. You may be asked how the third stage should be managed in the current pregnancy. This will be influenced by the aetiology of the problem in the last pregnancy.

DIABETES IN PREGNANCY ★★

DEFINITION

A clinical syndrome characterized by hyperglycaemia caused by relative insulin deficiency or reduced effectiveness of insulin.

The more recent classifications of diabetes into type 1 and type 2 disease may be unknown to some examiners, who are more familiar with the terms insulin dependent and non-insulin dependent. Gestational diabetes is defined as diabetes developing during pregnancy and resolving after delivery.

HISTORY

The main features to identify are the duration of the disease, its severity (in terms of peripheral vascular disease, retinopathy and nephropathy) and prepregnancy requirements for insulin and current dosage. Most diabetics will be on a twice-daily regimen, and you need to know how much of each type of insulin they take at each of these times.

If possible, identify the quality of glycaemic control around the time of conception. This relies on the patient being a 'complier' who might have planned her pregnancy. Well motivated diabetics tend to know their haemoglobin A_1 values, and this is worth asking about.

Ask what measures have been made during pregnancy to identify retinopathy and nephropathy. Ask directly about when the eyes were last formally examined.

The family history is occasionally relevant in type 1 diabetes, and should be asked about.

The history of the current pregnancy is important: menstrual upset is commoner in diabetics and the gestation at booking is important. Was a detailed ultrasound performed at 16–18 weeks? Was AFP screening performed?

It is worth including in your history a note of how the insulin requirements have increased. The name of the diabetic physician is also worth knowing, since they play a crucial role in the antenatal care.

EXAMINATION

Your general examination should address problems such as assessing vascular disease (the chances of finding a pregnant diabetic with significant vasculopathy is very small indeed, but nevertheless make a point of commenting on the normality of the capillary return). You must examine the retinas and comment on them. It is likely that you will know considerably more about the diabetic retina than your examiners. Pre-eclampsia is common in diabetics: check the blood pressure carefully.

Abdominal palpation is directed at identifying a macrosomic fetus or polyhydramnios. Alternatively, you may find no abnormality or even evidence of IUGR if the disease is poorly controlled and there is small vessel disease. Measure the abdominal girth and elicit or exclude a fluid thrill.

FACTFILE

1. Fetal anomaly is less common in women attending prepregnancy clinics for diabetics than those who do not attend.
2. HbA_1 levels of greater than 12% are associated with increased rates of fetal anomaly, particularly neural tube defect and cardiac disease.
3. Insulin requirements drop within 24 hours of delivery to almost prepregnancy levels.
4. Urinalysis is useless for monitoring diabetic control in pregnancy.

DISCUSSION POINTS

1. The normal physiology of glucose control is beloved of some people, and you ought to be familiar with both the pattern of normal renal clearance in pregnancy as well as the pattern of insulin secretion in pregnancy.

2. The criteria for normality of a glucose tolerance test and how you might perform such a test provide useful starting points for discussion, as do the value of screening the normal population for impaired glucose tolerance in pregnancy.

3. It is alarming how many students are unable to describe clearly how glucose tolerance tests are performed. Like asking someone to describe how you would obtain a midstream specimen of urine, it identifies those who have actually 'been around' and those who have not.

PREVIOUS FETAL LOSS/ABNORMALITY ★

DEFINITIONS

- **Abortion** The termination of a pregnancy before 24 weeks gestation which results in the expulsion of a fetus that shows no signs of life.
- **Stillbirth** The delivery after 24 weeks gestation of a fetus that shows no sign of life.
- **Early neonatal death** Death within 1 week of delivery of a live newborn, regardless of the gestational age at delivery.
- **Late neonatal death** Death between 1 and 4 weeks of a newborn, regardless of the gestational age at delivery.
- **Perinatally related infant death** Death of an infant between 4 weeks and 1 year of life from a cause that was perinatally related.

Principal causes

- Intrauterine growth restriction ★★★
- Fetal abnormality ★★
- Prematurity ★★★
- Infection ★★
- Maternal hypertension ★★★
- Maternal alloimmunization ★★
- Trauma ★
- Antepartum haemorrhage ★★★

HISTORY

The history taking should be directed at identifying the cause of the previous loss or the nature of the fetal abnormality. This may require even more sensitivity than you normally use. Identify the measures that have been taken to identify or exclude a recurrence of the problem.

EXAMINATION

Try to relate the findings to the causes of previous losses: for example, if the history is of previous preterm labour then think whether there is any finding you might make in the current pregnancy. An 'irritable' uterus at 29 weeks' gestation might in these circumstances be highly significant. Similarly, if you suspect that the fundus of the uterus feels unusual, perhaps there is a septate uterus or other malformation which might lead to premature delivery.

DISCUSSION POINTS

1. The classification of perinatal mortality is not standardized throughout the UK, but you should be able to describe the relative contributions that, for example, fetal abnormality and infection contribute. You should

know the perinatal mortality rate in the hospitals in which you have undertaken your obstetric attachment.

2. The management points involved in these cases relate first to the cause of the loss and secondly to the type of care that should be given in such cases. This can largely be psychological support. There is no harm in stressing that this should be part of the management plan.

RHESUS DISEASE ★

DEFINITION

A condition wherein maternal IgG class antibodies cause fetal haemolysis, most commonly because of previous maternal exposure to rhesus D antigen. Other antigens can cause fetal haemolysis, and many of the principles of the management of rhesus disease are common to other antigens.

HISTORY

Previous exposure is required in order for a woman to become isoimmunized. This is commonly from previous pregnancies, but earlier blood transfusion is a rare cause. Failure of prophylaxis, either administrative or true therapeutic failure, is becoming the most important cause of rhesus disease in the UK. Determine the likely sensitizing event. This will usually be a pregnancy, though a history of blood transfusion is important. Failure to administer anti-D prophylaxis following previous termination of pregnancy should not be forgotten. If the patient has undergone previous abortion, either spontaneous or induced, she should be aware of whether anti-D was given. If she is not, there may be a number of possible explanations (such as her poor memory), but nevertheless this is an important point to make to the examiners.

Check whether the patient is aware of the likely genotype of her partner. Useful questions relate to whether she has been told that the baby will definitely be affected (partner homozygous D) or if there is only a 50% chance (partner heterozygous). If you are lucky she may also be aware of the titre of antibody or quantitation.

The past obstetric history should be very clearly presented. Specifically, find out how badly affected previous babies were and at what gestations invasive investigations or treatments were begun. Find out what investigations relevant to the diagnosis have been made in the current pregnancy. If, for example, amniocentesis has already been performed, find out at what gestation. Fetal blood sampling may have been performed, either diagnostically or for the purposes of intravascular transfusion. The significance of the gestation at delivery and whether this was iatrogenic is worthy of emphasis, as is the duration of stay for the baby in the neonatal unit and the number of exchange transfusions (if the mother is aware of this).

EXAMINATION

Remember that isoimmunization is a disease of the fetus rather than of the mother, so general examination will usually be unremarkable. The one exception to this might be if the fetus is hydropic and polyhydramnios has developed, but this would be a very unusual case to be presented with in the examination situation. Nevertheless, take note of the clinical impression of the liquor volume.

1. 1% of rhesus negative women become isoimmunized during pregnancy. Antepartum administration of anti-D reduces this frequency to about 0.3%.
2. As rhesus D problems reduce, the incidence of other red cell antigens causing problems is increasing. These are Kell, anti-C, anti-c and anti-E. Other antigens may also cause fetal haemolysis, but are relatively rare.
3. 500 IU of anti-D covers a fetomaternal haemorrhage of 4 ml.

DISCUSSION POINTS

1. Discussion of the management of non-sensitized rhesus-negative women during pregnancy is as likely as a question on the management of rhesus disease.
2. The indications for and dosage of anti-D may be mentioned in connection with a number of cases. For example, if you present a case of antepartum haemorrhage in a rhesus-negative woman you must mention the need for anti-D.

AN A–Z IN OBSTETRICS AND GYNAECOLOGY

QUESTIONS

ABORTION

A1 What are the legal requirements that must be fulfilled prior to termination of pregnancy in the UK?

ADENOMYOSIS

A2 What are the clinical features of adenomyosis?

A3 How do you diagnose adenomyosis?

ALPHA-FETOPROTEIN (AFP)

A4 What is the sensitivity and specificity of maternal screening using AFP alone for neural tube defect?

AMNIOCENTESIS

A5 What is the procedure-related abortion rate following amniocentesis?

ANTEPARTUM HAEMORRHAGE

A6 Define antepartum haemorrhage. What are the principal causes?

ANTI-D

A7 When should anti-D be administered?

ASTHMA

A8 What is the effect of pregnancy on asthma?

ASYMPTOMATIC BACTERIURIA

A9 What is meant by the term asymptomatic bacteriuria?

BIOPHYSICAL PROFILE SCORING

B1 What are the components of the biophysical scoring system?

BISHOP SCORE

B2 What are the components of the Bishop score?

CA125

C1 In what circumstances is CA125 elevated?

CARDIOTOCOGRAPHY (CTG)

C2 What is meant by a 'reactive' CTG?

CERVICAL CERCLAGE

C3 At what gestation should cerclage be performed?

CHORION VILLUS SAMPLING (CVS)

C4 What is the abortion rate following CVS?

CYSTOCOELE

C5 What risk factors are implicated in development of cystocoele?

ECLAMPSIA

E1 Which drug would you use to control convulsions in an eclamptic woman at 37 weeks' gestation?

ENDOMETRIAL BIOPSY

E2 How might endometrial biopsies be obtained?

FETAL ABNORMALITY

F1 What is the incidence of neural tube defect in the UK?

FIBROIDS IN GYNAECOLOGY

F2 What is the incidence of malignant change in leiomyomata?

FIBROIDS IN OBSTETRICS

F3 How might fibroids present in obstetric practice?

FORCEPS

F4 What conditions must be met before forceps should be used to expedite delivery?

GALACTORRHOEA

G1 What are the possible causes of galactorrhoea?

GENUINE STRESS INCONTINENCE

G2 Define the term genuine stress incontinence.

GLUCOSE TOLERANCE TESTING

G3 What are the criteria for impaired glucose tolerance?

GONORRHOEA

G4 What are the clinical features of gonorrhoea in the female?

G5 Should women with gonorrhoea be compulsorily tested for HIV infection?

HEART DISEASE

H1 What is the New York Heart Association classification of heart disease, and is it relevant to pregnancy?

HIRSUTISM

H2 Define hirsutism.

HORMONE REPLACEMENT THERAPY (HRT)

H3 By what routes may HRT be administered?

INDUCTION OF LABOUR

I1 What are the indications for induction of labour?

INFERTILITY

I2 What is the incidence of infertility in the general population?

INTRAUTERINE CONTRACEPTIVE DEVICE (IUCD)

I3 What are the complications of IUCD use?

IRON SUPPLEMENTATION IN PREGNANCY

I4 What is the normal daily dietary requirement for iron in pregnancy?

LACTATION

L1 What methods of lactation suppression are used in your hospital, and which women should routinely receive such treatment?

MATERNAL AGE

M1 What is the effect of increasing maternal age on perinatal mortality?

MATERNAL MORTALITY

M2 What are the commonest causes of death in the most recent confidential enquiries into maternal deaths in the UK?

MIDSTREAM SPECIMEN OF URINE (MSSU)

M3 How would you instruct a woman to provide an uncontaminated midstream specimen?

NEURAL TUBE DEFECT

N1 Does fetal limb movement *in utero* predict handicap in cases of spina bifida?

OVARIAN CYSTS

O1 What complications may ovarian cysts undergo?

OVARIAN TUMOURS

O2 Classify ovarian tumours.

OXYTOCIN

O3 What is the pharmacology of oxytocin?

PERINATAL DEATH

P1 What investigations should be performed following a perinatal loss?

PFANNENSTIEL

P2 Who was Pfannenstiel?

POLYCYSTIC OVARY SYNDROME (PCOS)

P3 What are the diagnostic criteria for PCOS?

POLYHYDRAMNIOS

P4 What are the causes of polyhydramnios?

POSTCOITAL CONTRACEPTION

P5 What methods of postcoital contraception are available?

POSTMENOPAUSAL BLEEDING

P6 Define postmenopausal bleeding.

POSTPARTUM HAEMORRHAGE

P7 Define secondary postpartum haemorrhage.

PRE-ECLAMPSIA

P8 What is pre-eclampsia?

PREMATURE RUPTURE OF THE MEMBRANES

P9 What is the difference between premature rupture of the membranes and preterm rupture of the membranes?

PREMENSTRUAL SYNDROME (PMS)

P10 What is PMS?

PRIMARY AMENORRHOEA

P11 What is the commonest cause of primary amenorrhoea?

QUICKENING

Q1 When does quickening occur in a multigravida?

RECURRENT ABORTION

R1 Define recurrent abortion.

ROUTINE ANTENATAL CARE

R2 What is the pattern of antenatal care that should be provided for a low-risk primigravida?

SICKLE CELL DISEASE

S1 Which patients should be screened for sickle cell trait?

STERILIZATION

S2 What is the failure rate of laparoscopic sterilization using falope rings?

SYPHILIS

S3 When should women be screened for syphilis?

TERATOGENESIS

T1 Which drugs are unequivocally associated with teratogenesis?

THALASSAEMIA

T2 What types of thalassaemia are of importance to obstetricians?

THIRD STAGE OF LABOUR

T3 Describe the management of the normal third stage of labour.

TRIPLET PREGNANCY

T4 What is the natural incidence of triplet pregnancy?

UNSTABLE LIE

U1 What are the common causes of unstable lie?

URINARY INCONTINENCE

U2 What is incontinence?

URODYNAMICS

U3 What is meant by the term urodynamic assessment?

UTEROVAGINAL PROLAPSE

U4 What types of uterovaginal prolapse do you know?

VAGINAL DISCHARGE

V1 What are the common causes of vaginal discharge?

VENTOUSE DELIVERY

V2 What conditions must be met before a ventouse delivery is undertaken?

VESICOVAGINAL FISTULA

V3 What are the causes of vesicovaginal fistula?

VULVAL DISEASE

V4 Classify vulval epithelial disorders.

V5 Does vulval intraepithelial neoplasia have a viral aetiology?

WARTS

W1 What is the topical treatment of choice for vulval warts?

WEIGHING DURING ANTENATAL VISITS

W2 What is the normal weight gain in pregnancy?

X-RAYS

X1 What was the 10-day rule?

ZOONOSIS

Z1 Which foodstuffs are associated with listeria and toxoplasma?

ZYGOSITY

Z2 What is the likely zygosity of triplets resulting from IVF?

ANSWERS

A1 1. To save the mother's life

2. To prevent grave permanent injury to the mother's physical or mental health

3. If less than 24 weeks, termination may be performed to avoid injury to the physical or mental health of the mother or to avoid injury to the physical or mental health of the existing child(ren)

4. If the child is likely to be severely physically or mentally handicapped.

A2 Painful heavy periods.

A3 Diagnosis is made on examination of a hysterectomy specimen.

A4   AFP screening will detect almost all cases of anencephaly and around 85–90% of cases of spina bifida. In pregnancies associated with otherwise unexplained elevated AFP only 1 in 10 to 1 in 15 will actually have a neural tube defect.

A5   0.5%.

A6   Bleeding from the genital tract from 24 weeks gestation until delivery of the fetus. The principal causes are placental abruption and placenta praevia.

A7   Anti-D should be given to all rhesus-negative women who are not already rhesus isoimmunized and who:
- have a threatened abortion
- undergo termination of pregnancy
- miscarry
- have antepartum haemorrhage
- undergo external cephalic version
- experience blunt abdominal trauma
- undergo amniocentesis or chorion villus sampling
- deliver a baby whose blood group is unknown
- deliver a baby who is known to be rhesus positive.

A8   The majority of women experience no change in symptoms. In one-third, however, the condition improves and in one-fifth it deteriorates.

A9   A bacterial count of 100 000 bacteria per ml in a midstream specimen of urine in the absence of symptoms.

B1   Fetal body movement, fetal breathing movement, fetal tone, liquor volume and cardiotocography.

B2   Dilatation, length, consistency and position of the cervix and station of the presenting part.

C1   CA125 is elevated in cases of ovarian cancer, endometriosis, fibroids and non-gynaecological conditions such as colonic cancer.

C2 A CTG is reactive if it shows two accelerations of at least 15 beats per minute lasting at least 15 seconds in a 20-minute monitoring period.

C3 Electively at 12–16 weeks gestation.

C4 The excess loss rate over the risk of spontaneous abortion is around 1%.

C5 High parity, obesity, chronic cough, obstetric trauma.

E1 Magnesium sulphate.

E2 Endometrial aspiration by Vabra technique or Pipelle aspirator, diagnostic curettage.

F1 2–3 per 1000. The incidence is higher in the north and west and lower in the south and east.

F2 Less than 0.5%.

F3 Large-for-dates uterus, malpresentation, spontaneous abortion, preterm labour and, less commonly, obstructed labour and pain with red degeneration.

F4 There must be a valid indication, the cervix must be fully dilated, the position must be known, there must be no evidence of disproportion and the bladder must be empty. Ideally there should be adequate analgesia/anaesthesia. This last condition may not necessarily be achievable if there is marked fetal distress.

G1 Lactation! Drugs causing hyperprolactinaemia, e.g. cimetidine, phenothiazines. Prolactinoma.

G2 Involuntary leakage of urine when the intravesical pressure exceeds the urethral closure pressure in the absence of detrusor activity.

G3 Fasting glucose of less than 8 mM/l and a 2-hour value between 8 and 11 mM/l.

G4 Often none, but may present as acute pelvic inflammatory disease.

G5 No.

H1 Class 1 have no functional limitation. Class 2 have slight limitation of physical activity. Class 3 patients experience a marked limitation of physical activity but are comfortable at rest. Class 4 have symptoms present at rest and inability to perform any physical activity without discomfort. The classification is valid in pregnancy, but classes 3 and 4 are rarely seen in the UK.

H2 The subjective assessment of the patient (or her acquaintances!) that she has excessive hair in an abnormal site.

H3 Oral, subcutaneous implant, topical (patch or gel).

I1 Induction of labour is indicated when the risks to mother or fetus of continuation of the pregnancy exceed the dangers of the induction process or prematurity. Examples in the maternal interest include pre-eclampsia, and in the fetal interest IUGR would be the classic example.

I2 15%.

I3 The commonest is menorrhagia. Other complications relate to aspects of insertion, such as the introduction of infection or perforation of the uterus.

I4 100 mg.

L1 Breast binding is the simplest effective method. Women who have experienced perinatal loss should receive help with suppression of lactation. In this group of women this may include the use of bromocriptine.

M1 Perinatal mortality is greatest at the extremes of the reproductive age groups. The perinatal mortality rate in teenagers is 25% greater than in women between 20 and 30. In women over 30 the risk is 15% greater than in this group.

M2 Hypertensive disorders, pulmonary embolism and haemorrhage.

M3 The vulva should be wiped with a clean cloth from the clitoris posteriorly. Soap and disinfectants should not be used. She should start passing urine and during this collect the urine in an appropriate sterile container which is placed into the urine stream. When enough has been collected this is removed from the urine stream and put aside for investigation.

N1 No.

O1 Haemorrhage, torsion, rupture and infection.

O2 • Epithelial tumours, e.g. mucinous cystadenoma
• Sex cord gonadal tumours e.g .granulosa tumours
• Germ cell tumours, e.g. teratomas
• Miscellaneous, e.g. lymphoma
• Secondary, e.g. Krukenberg.

O3 Oxytocin acts through stimulation of oxytocin receptors in the uterus to produce calcium-mediated contractions.

P1 • Viral titres for fetotoxic organisms, e.g. toxoplasma
• Red cell antibodies
• Lupus anticoagulant and anticardiolipin antibodies
• Postmortem of the baby, including karyotype
• Kleihauer test.

P2 A German gynaecologist who lived 1862–1909. The transverse suprapubic incision he developed for pelvic surgery now carries his name.

P3 *Biochemical:* LH/FSH ratio of 3 or greater

Ultrasound: classic appearance of enlarged ovaries with small cysts seen peripherally in the ovary.

P4 *Maternal:* diabetes

Fetal: Neural tube defect, anterior abdominal wall defect, oesophageal atresia, hydrops fetalis, Pierre Robin syndrome

Placental: Haemangioma.

P5 IUCD, high-dose oestrogen in the form of 50 μg of ethinyl oestradiol with levonorgestrel as two tablets on two occasions 12 hours apart.

P6 Bleeding from the genital tract 1 or more years after the menopause.

P7 Excessive vaginal blood loss from 24 hours after delivery until 6 weeks later. (The volume lost is not part of the definition.)

P8 Pre-eclampsia is a condition of unknown aetiology occurring usually in the second half of pregnancy, usually in primigravidas, and characterized by hypertension, proteinuria and oedema.

P9 In the UK there is generally considered to be no difference. In North America the same term is used to describe rupture of the membranes before labour is established, regardless of the gestational age.

P10 A condition characterized by cyclical variation in symptoms, which improve after the onset of menstruation.

P11 Constitutional delay.

Q1 Fifteen to 19 weeks on average.

R1 Three or more consecutive spontaneous abortions.

R2 This varies between different centres and among obstetricians.

S1 Black women and women with abnormal blood indices.

S2 Between 1 in 500 and 1 in 1000 operations.

S3 All women are screened in early pregnancy and following a history of (possible) exposure or symptoms.

T1 The chief culprits are thalidomide, bisphosphonates, all anticonvulsants.

T2 All types!

T3 The third stage of labour is usually managed 'actively' by administration of syntometrine with delivery of the anterior shoulder (in a singleton pregnancy). The placenta is delivered following signs of separation by controlled cord traction.

T4 1 in 6400 pregnancies.

U1 Polyhydramnios, high parity.

U2 The term 'urinary incontinence' describes involuntary loss of urine and gives no indication of aetiology.

U3 Urodynamic assessment describes a range of investigations of the urinary tract, including cystoscopy and intravenous urography, but is commonly used to mean cystometry.

U4 Cystocoele, rectocoele, enterocoele, urethrocoele and the three degrees of uterine prolapse.

V1 Candidal and trichomonal vaginitis, bacterial vaginosis and physiological.

V2 The same as for forceps delivery but in extreme circumstances (uncommon in the UK) may be used before full dilatation.

V3 Trauma (including obstetric), iatrogenic, radiation and malignancy (usually of the cervix).

V4 Non-neoplastic disorders, i.e. lichen sclerosus, squamous cell hyperplasia and other dermatoses. Vulval intraepithelial neoplasia, which is subdivided into squamous and non-squamous VIN. Carcinoma.

V5 The answer to this question remains unclear.

W1 Podophyllin paint.

W2 The average gain is 12.5 kg, but the range of weight gain in normal pregnancies is very wide.

X1 Women in the reproductive age group should undergo X-rays within 10 days of the first day of their last menstrual period.

Z1 Listeria infection is associated with soft cheeses and paté. Toxoplasma is associated with incompletely cooked meat products.

Z2 Trizygotic.

PAEDIATRICS

HISTORY AND EXAMINATION IN PAEDIATRICS

The clinical examination in paediatrics differs from the others in many respects. The first of these is that you must establish a relationship with a child or infant, as well as with the parents and examiners. Many medical schools have abandoned long cases in paediatrics and replaced them with a series of short cases. This means that you must establish your relationship with the patient very quickly, since you will still need to take a history as well as perform competent clinical examination and elicit clinical signs.

As with the other disciplines there is no substitute for previous experience. If you have not been in the wards and cannot examine a child or are intimidated by them, you do not deserve to pass. You must have practised communicating with children before the exams. Your results will be better if you know basic facts and can demonstrate that you do not have every 5-year-old running away from you, than if you know every obscure paediatric syndrome but every child you see hides under mother's coat until you have gone away!

At this point it is worth pointing out that your demeanour is best directed at the patient. Modern paediatric wards are fairly informal places, and much has been written about how doctors are perceived by children. Your approach to the examiners must always be formal, but you can approach the child, through his or her parents, in an informal fashion.

EQUIPMENT

You will already possess a stethoscope and tendon hammer and perhaps even your own ophthalmoscope. In paediatrics it is more important to possess a tape measure than a tendon hammer. A torch is equally important. In order to impress the examiners it is worth bringing some children's bricks or toys to attract the child's attention and perform developmental assessment if needed. Borrow these if necessary.

HISTORY TAKING

When you take the history a parent will often be available. The important thing here is never to approach the child directly. You must demonstrate to the child that his or her parent is comfortable with you and that you are no kind of threat. With younger children you should avoid starting off by asking direct questions of the child, since this can result in a clam-like attitude on their part. The parent will then only respond to the anxieties provoked in their child, so you have lost their confidence too. This remains a good rule even with older children.

When you take the history this must be from the very beginning, i.e. the history of the pregnancy. Particular attention should be paid to the occurrence of any complications during the pregnancy, the mode of delivery and, crucially, the gestational age at delivery. Admission to a neonatal unit and duration of stay is also important.

A developmental history should be taken and may even be the point of one of the cases. You should know how to do this already, but in essence the milestones of smiling, standing, independent walking and acquisition of hand skills should be documented. Remember always to relate this to gestationally adjusted age and not age from birth. It follows that you must know the normal age of reaching these milestones.

Nutrition is important and you should identify the quality and quantity of the child's eating pattern. This applies to infant feeding as well the older child, and you should certainly know whether the baby was breastfed or not. In connection with this you must be familiar with the growth charts used in paediatrics. If you are presented with one and do not have a clue about the meanings of centile values and how the charts are used (including correction for gestational age) then you create a very poor impression, since these are fundamental in paediatric practice.

Family history is important in this connection, as parental size may be important. Other aspects of the family history are as important as in any other field, but there are certain clues that should be sought and the behaviour and health of siblings are important. There may be other relatives with related problems. These may be forgotten by parents, and it is worth asking if any relatives had health problems in childhood, attended special schools or had special educational needs.

Social history is of obvious importance, but specific enquiry should be made about whether the parents smoke. This requires tact and caution: you should not alienate the parents, on whom you rely for further information.

In older children ask about school absence and performance.

You should have mastered the other aspects of history taking, but their application in paediatrics requires practice.

EXAMINATION

Before you begin to examine the patient you must already have established a relationship with both parent – usually the mother – and child. Remember to smile. This is so basic, but very difficult if you yourself are feeling a little strained because of the examination. Once again, practice and familiarity with examining children should help. Ask the mother if you may examine her child. The child must realise that this stranger is not a threat and that mother agrees to the examination. Once you have established this, speak to the child. This is by no means easy, and it is important to take note of the child's response. A child who is very shy may be so naturally, or be frightened by you, or hospitals, or by adults generally. This may be a clue to significant underlying problems and may be worthy of later comment. Similarly an overly affectionate child, looking for love and attention, may also be expressing underlying problems.

Be nice to the patient. This little person is probably a lot more anxious than you are and really does not care about your worries. If you are kind to the child in the finals you will keep your examiners happy even if you do not know the minutiae. Always remember this.

Finally, if you are seeing more than one patient in the exam, for example between short cases, you must remember to wash your hands between patients unless you are instructed to the contrary.

GENERAL PHYSICAL EXAMINATION

There are a few general points that you should have reached before you examine the child formally. While you have been taking the history you should already have formed an impression of whether the child has any dysmorphic features. These may be obvious, as in Down syndrome. Less immediately obvious, at least at the outset, will be features such as whether the head is proportionate in size to the trunk.

You will know the child's age, chronological and gestationally adjusted, and you should know if he or she is small for his or her age. This depends on your knowledge of the normal range of size for children of a given age. Failure to identify a significant discrepancy in size for age is a sure indication to the examiners that your presence on the wards has been less than colossal.

Take note of the child's response to you and the other adults. Is he or she withdrawn or suspicious?

When you begin the examination always ask for the mother's help to undress the child – not to restrain but to encourage the child (if possible). It is important to mention that there is no absolutely correct way to perform a physical examination in paediatrics. Much of the examination might be made in an opportunistic fashion. A systematic approach or a 'top to tail' approach may be attempted, but success with either depends on a huge number of variables. Your capacity to adapt will again indicate to the examiners that you are not new to the difficulties of examining children.

It is fair to say that you will rarely be asked to perform a detailed general examination. It is more likely that you will be instructed to listen to or examine the child's chest. You should still take note of all the other clues mentioned above.

For clarity of layout the examination style presented will follow a systematic approach.

Cardiovascular system

Look for the obvious things, such as clubbing and cyanosis. Distinguish peripheral from central cyanosis. Tachypnoea may also be a more obvious sign of cardiac disease than in the adult.

Check both arm pulses: one absent radial pulse is distinctly possible in a child who has undergone surgery for Fallot's tetralogy. Similarly feel the femoral pulses: absent or poor-quality femoral pulses raises the possibility of coarctation of the aorta. Generally you will not be asked to check the blood pressure, but you should know generalities about the automatic blood pressure monitors that are used so much in paediatrics.

Palpate the chest before auscultation. Cardiac thrills are often pronounced in children and the site of the apex beat must be identified. Do not get too excited about the characteristics of any murmurs. You should know the basics, so do try to identify systolic or diastolic murmurs but do not panic if it all sounds very complicated. Paediatric cardiologists use echocardiography, so they obviously find some of the sounds confusing! You should know how to grade a murmur, however.

Remember that you may be asked to examine a normal child. Flow murmurs are common!

Respiratory system

Make a point of counting the respiratory rate and identifying intercostal and sternal recession. As in cardiac disease, you should identify clubbing if present. It is unlikely that you will see a case such as severe asthma, but do remember that the asthmatic child without a wheeze who cannot talk is probably very much sicker than a wheezy talker.

In children younger than 1 year old percussion of the chest is not very helpful and may frighten the child. In older children it may be helpful, Auscultation of the chest is usually helpful, but possibly less so in infants. You should be aware of how to measure peak expiratory flow using Wright's peak flow meter. You should also be familiar with the various types of inhalers, spacer devices and nebulizers.

The observation that a child is receiving oxygen by nasal cannula is worth comment, and if in addition the child has a hyperinflated chest, is less than a year old and is small, should ring an alarm bell that says this child is a survivor of prematurity with bronchopulmonary dysplasia.

Abdominal examination

Treat the paediatric abdomen with gentleness. Cold hands and too firm an initial touch will result in a disgruntled and uncooperative patient. Do not hurry this bit of the examination. Talk to the child gently and quietly while you examine. This also ensures that you are looking at the child's face rather than the abdomen as you palpate, and this is important. The initial palpation must be very superficial in every sense, since the spleen in particular can be readily felt if enlarged. Roll the child on to his or her right side to further increase the prospects of identifying a splenic problem. Remember to feel for the lower border of the liver and, if appropriate, percuss for the upper limit.

Once confidence is established (both yours and the child's) you can palpate more deeply.

Ticklish children are a problem, but often the examiners will recognize this and if you are lucky direct you to something else.

If you think there is ascites then involve the examiner or parent in helping you elicit a fluid thrill.

Never ever forget to examine the hernial orifices. This might be the point of the whole exam, so do not forget.

You should also make an attempt to examine the genitalia (but only in the presence of the parents or examiners). If the child is dressed you should say, for example, that you would like to remove the nappy. This in itself might be all the examiners want to hear and that may not even ask you to continue, but do mention it.

Examination of the skin

Any rashes in paediatric exams are likely to be eczema, psoriasis or possibly Henoch–Schönlein purpura. The infectious causes are very unlikely, since most paediatricians do not want rip-roaring chickenpox going through their wards. The one 'infectious' condition you might see is scabies, so remember to examine the feet and hands carefully.

You might occasionally see a case of Stevens–Johnson syndrome, so try to obtain a drug history if possible.

Limbs

You may be asked to examine the limbs. This is difficult, since if you have no history it may be uncertain whether the problem is an orthopaedic one, such as Perthe's disease, neurological, such as spina bifida (always examine the back), or an arthritis.

If the patient is old enough then try to assess the gait. You should know how to measure the limbs and check both for assymetry in size, but also for muscle wasting.

Isolated arthritis is a possible but unlikely case. Check for joint effusions.

The central nervous system

This is so interwoven with developmental assessment and examination of the limbs that you may already have reached a neurological diagnosis. First, take note of the size of the head and determine whether it is in proportion to the body. Measure the occipitofrontal circumference.

Neurological conditions in paediatrics can be complex, but the examiners do not want or expect you to identify obscure syndromes. Make all the relevant observations, but if you are unable to identify a common aetiology then do not panic.

Assess tone. You should recognize increased or decreased tone.

Assess power. Be sensible: if the child can walk without any problem then it is unlikely that there is any significant loss of power in the lower limbs.

In younger children you must be able to demonstrate primitive reflexes and know when they disappear. In older children clonus and mature reflexes should be elicited. The plantar reflex requires some sensitivity in use in children.

Examination of the eyes is important. Look particularly for squint and know the cover test. Using an ophthalmoscope can be challenging in paediatrics. The examiners will not expect you to identify any obscure problems, but you should appear confident in the use of this instrument. Once again practice and familiarity are the keys. Do not battle with the child to examine the fundi. If you must, then solicit the aid of the parents, or even the examiners. Do not hold the child's head still yourself. This may be frightening for the child and indeed the parents. Be flexible: you may only have the opportunity for a quick glimpse, but make use of it.

Cataracts would be an unlikely finding, but you should look for these as well as any obvious nystagmus.

If you are asked to examine the eyes then the odds are high that you will be asked about the nerves and muscles involved in eye movement. If you have not read this recently and do not remember them, then do so now!

Developmental assessment

It is very likely that you will be asked to perform a developmental assessment on any child. It is important to be aware that this does not necessarily mean that there is anything actually wrong with the child. Healthy children may take part in the examination.

Usually in such a case the patient will be 3 years old or younger. You will be asked to assess developmental age. This might provoke a question such as 'Why is this 3-year-old child performing at a 15-month level?'

Try to be logical in your assessment: if the child is sitting down and playing with a toy then it is time-wasting to talk about testing for appropriate smiling responses or head control and primitive reflexes.

If the child is not playing then use any (safe) articles lying around. If you have seen the child demonstrate pincer grasp during play then do not repeat this. You might not get the child to perform for you! Obviously a lot of developmental assessment is done fortuitously while watching the child.

Make note of the major areas: fine and gross motor skills can be assessed at play; vision and hand coordination likewise. Hearing and language may have to be more formally tested, so have a system for doing this. Social development can be difficult to determine in the context of a hospital, and also of a clinical examination such as the finals. A child who is obviously mixing with other children on the ward is easier to assess in this regard than the shy or withdrawn child, and this may be worth commenting upon to the examiners.

THE CASES

In contrast with the other final examination disciplines it is not as readily possible to present definitions or presentation of cases by symptomatology. A number of different conditions may present with a common range of symptoms. A history may be impossible to obtain and may appear to conflict with other clinical evidence. For example, you may be presented with a child who looks wasted and is failing to thrive but whose mother says the child is well and eats voraciously. This of course should raise clinical suspicions, but can be difficult for you to deal with during a clinical examination.

It is worth commenting that it would be quite unusual, though not impossible, to be presented with a newborn baby. Similarly, think of how likely certain conditions are to come up if you are sitting the exam during the spring or summer months: although you should know all about bronchiolitis, the chance of getting a case between May and July is negligible.

CARDIAC DISEASE ★★★★★

The two principal types of cardiac disease are cyanotic and acyanotic. Cyanotic disease is most commonly Fallot's tetralogy (★★★★) or transposition of the great vessels (★★★★). It is unlikely that you would see one of the other causes of cyanosis.

Symptoms as reported by parents are very important. Has the cyanosis been present from birth? Have there been feeding problems and colour changes with feeding? Parents may think that previous surgery is so obvious that they do not mention it to you, so be very clear about this aspect of the history.

On examination you want to identify whether there is cyanosis. If there is, then carefully distinguish between central and peripheral cyanosis. This is important both clinically and in the exam. Feel both radial arteries, especially if there is a history of previous surgery. Feel the femoral pulses. If you have to remove or move underwear to do this then enlist the help of the parents.

Palpate the chest for thrills and for the apex beat, since these can be more pronounced in children than in adults.

Another difference to be aware of is that children in cardiac failure do not usually have peripheral oedema but may well have more obvious liver enlargement.

Look for 'syndromes': trisomy 21 and trisomy 18 are both associated with complex cardiac lesions. Turner's syndrome is associated with coarctation and aortic stenosis.

FACTFILE

1. The commonest causes of acyanotic heart disease are ventricular septal defect, atrial septal defect, patent ductus arteriosus, pulmonary stenosis, aortic stenosis and coarctation of the aorta.
2. Around 12% of children with congenital cardiac problems have more than one heart defect.
3. Rheumatic heart disease is now rare in western practice, but may be seen in immigrant communities.

DISCUSSION POINTS

1. The investigations that might be undertaken in paediatric cardiology include echocardiography and Doppler examination of the vessels and flow across the valves. You need not know about these in detail, but should be familiar with the principles.

2. It is important to know the principles behind antibiotic prophylaxis for children with cardiac disease. Similarly, the management of subacute bacterial endocarditis should be familiar to you.
3. Newer minimally invasive techniques of treating obstructive cardiac disease are becoming established and you may be asked about these.
4. Many heart murmurs are innocent in children, and you might be asked what advice you would give the parents of a child with such a finding.

DEVELOPMENTAL DELAY ★★★★★

A child who fails to reach the milestones in the major developmental areas within the normal range is said to exhibit developmental delay. The causes are numerous but, as previously discussed, the birth and family history are particularly important. Social interaction is important, and developmental delay may result from poor stimulation and can result in a child who is clearly failing to thrive.

It is worth repeating that you must know the major milestones. If you think that unintelligible babble is appropriate for a 26-month-old child then you have a problem, since the examiners will think that you and the child share some characteristics – i.e. your contribution may be unintelligible babble to them!

If possible, your general examination should be linked with the developmental assessment, and this highlights that a lot of paediatric examination technique is opportunistic.

DISCUSSION POINTS

1. Environmental effects on childhood development are currently being emphasized in both the lay and the medical literature. You may be asked to comment on which aspect of the environment is the greatest contributor to developmental delay.

2. What single aspect of medical care may improve the outcome in developmental delay?

3. The interaction of the child with other members of the family and family stress may promote problems with development. How might these be alleviated?

4. It is very important to be aware of and able to discuss, at least superficially, the many different disciplines involved in the care of the handicapped child. Neurologists, ophthalmologists, psychologists and many therapists will contribute to the care of these children, as well as paediatricians.

NEUROLOGICAL DISORDERS ★★★★★

The cases that might present under this heading are variable. The most likely are cerebral palsy ★★★★★ or spina bifida ★★. You may be presented with an epileptic child, though this is unlikely. In practical terms it may be easier for exam organizers to find a child admitted with febrile convulsions.

The history should be relatively straightforward. Although the vast majority of cerebral palsy is unrelated to intrapartum events, you must obtain a comprehensive birth history. A history of prematurity and prolonged early hospitalization is very important. You should know the different types of cerebral palsy, e.g. hemiplegic, diplegic and so on.

The family and social history is important in these cases. How is the family as a whole coping? The educational needs of the child should be discussed and any plans the parents have formed outlined.

Your examination should determine the degree of handicap. If you are asked to examine a child whose head looks disproportionately large, then do remember that hydrocephalus still occurs. When you examine such a child make sure to check the site of the shunt. It is also worth measuring the parental head size if possible.

Assess the degree of the child's mobility.

THE SCRAWNY/SMALL CHILD ★★★★★

You may be presented with a child who is failing to thrive. Your history should identify any obvious genetic points and the child's initial development. The principal points during examination relate to whether the child is appropriately nourished and proportionately small. This kind of child, may represent a constitutionally small child, whereas the findings of muscle wasting with a distended abdomen suggest an organic problem.

In a little girl remember the possibility of Turner's syndrome. Endocrine problems such as growth hormone deficiency and hypothyroidism are not common, but the examiners will be happy to discuss these treatable problems.

Social history is very important in these children, as failure to thrive is not infrequently associated with neglect.

It is essential to correlate your findings to growth charts. If you are presented with a small child and have not used the appropriate growth charts or suggested their use you will fail (or deserve to). Disproportionate smallness may be due to achondroplasia, so assess long bone length.

FACTFILE

1. In a Newcastle community study of 98 children below the third centile for height there were six chromosomal problems, one case each of cystic fibrosis, chronic renal failure, cyanotic congenital cardiac disease growth, hormone deficiency and Hurler's syndrome, and four defined as mental handicap.
2. Coeliac disease is a rare but recognized cause of small stature. The incidence appears to be reducing, possibly owing to a reduction in childhood exposure to dietary allergens.
3. Congenital hypothyroidism should be excluded by the introduction of neonatal screening, so the majority of hypothyroid cases are juveniles.
4. Birth length is doubled at age 4 and trebled by the age of 13.

DISCUSSION POINTS

1. You will be expected to be familiar with the use of growth charts and how they are used.
2. The role of the environment in childhood growth and development is important and may well be discussed.

3. The investigation of the small child is a reasonable topic, but since it can appear all-embracing it is important to have a clear idea of what is involved and not to jump to invasive tests too early.

THE BREATHLESS CHILD ★★★★

Breathlessness may be a factor in many different paediatric problems. These can be infectious, such as bronchiolitis (★★★, but remember this is seasonal), environmental/ genetic, such as asthma (★★★★★), or genetic, such as cystic fibrosis (★★★★).

Heart defects may also present with breathlessness.

The history should be directed towards identifying the most likely underlying problem, such as a genetic or family history, as in cystic fibrosis, or a family history of atopy. Social history is important. Establish whether the parents smoke. This can be difficult since, as previously mentioned, you must try not to alienate the parents.

Drug history is important. If the child uses inhalers try to identify how suitable this is for a child of his or her age. Some children are given standard inhalers when patient-triggered or spacer devices would be much more effective. Find out if prophylactic treatment is being given and get some idea of compliance (on the part of either the child or the parent).

On examination assess growth. All children with severe underlying disease are likely to have some impairment of growth. This is especially likely in children with cystic fibrosis. Look for other signs: clubbing may be seen.

FACTFILE

1. 13% of children with cystic fibrosis will not present until they are 5 years old or older.
2. Half of all children with cystic fibrosis will present before 6 months of age. Most will present with respiratory illness or failure to thrive because of malabsorption.
3. Acute bronchiolitis is usually a winter disease, and implicated viruses include parainfluenza, rhino and adenoviruses, although the respiratory syncytial virus is the best-remembered one.
4. The incidence of asthma is increasing dramatically. Air pollution is not the only cause, but environmental factors do appear to be very significant.

DISCUSSION POINTS

1. You may be asked about the different types of inhaler that might be used in children.
2. The difference between the treatment of acute asthma and ongoing management with maintenance is sometimes blurred in difficult cases, but you should be able to distinguish what you mean by these terms.
3. Peak flow meters are important in assessing the older child. Know how to use one. A useful test for examiners is to ask candidates how they would instruct a child to use a peak flow meter. If you have not 'been around' this can be tricky.

DYSMORPHISM ★★★★

In large teaching hospitals in particular, medical students leave paediatrics with the impression that the specialty is preoccupied with syndromes. This is not true, but there are a number of syndromes with which you should be familiar. These are Down syndrome (★★★★★), Edward syndrome (★), Turner's syndrome (★★★) and Klinefelter's syndrome (★).

There are other syndromes that you may see during teaching. A small hint is that if they are rare and chronic with prolonged hospitalization, you may see the same child in the exam!

In your history and examination you should aim to identify the specific abnormalities the child has. Even if you have the greatest mental blank and cannot remember the common name of trisomy 21, you should comment on developmental delay, the presence of a heart defect, floppiness and characteristic facies.

Put another way, the examiners will not care too much if you cannot remember Treacher–Collins syndrome if you can summarize the clinical features the patient presents.

Your history should identify what medical, social, family and educational problems the family is experiencing in bringing up their child. If you have time it is worth identifying the effects, if any, on any siblings.

LUMPS AND BUMPS ★★★★

Many medical schools also include paediatric surgical cases in the finals. You may be asked to examine the abdomen. Make a point of identifying organomegaly (★★★★★). Hernial (★★★★★) orifices must be checked. Umbilical hernias (★★★★) are very common, though, and you should know that they only very rarely require surgery. Consequently, if presented with such a case and you have the opportunity, try to find out whether there is any other reason for the child being in hospital. This may get you some Brownie points.

Groin hernias in boys are commonly inguinal, but in girls they may also be femoral.

You should recognise hydrocoeles (★★★★★) and also be aware of the difference between maldescent and undescent of the testes. Once again, the need for the cooperation of parents in this aspect of the examination cannot be over-emphasized.

SKIN PROBLEMS ★★★★

You may be asked to examine a rash or skin lesion, and your description should use the standard dermatological terms of papular, macular, erythematous etc. At the end of your description you should be able to reach some kind of diagnosis, the commonest of which are ammoniacal dermatitis (★★★★), atopic eczema (★★★★★) and the various types of naevus (★★★★★). Psoriasis (★★) may also be seen.

Infectious causes may also be seen, so look between the fingers and on the feet for scabies and warts. Head lice have not been eradicated so do look, just in case. Psoriasis may also be present on the scalp, and is important to comment upon if so.

History should identify the aetiological factors. Atopy is important and a specific family history should be sought. Similarly, any obvious allergens should be identified if possible.

PAINFUL JOINT(S) ★★

Painful swollen joints are more likely to be rheumatic in origin than septic. Rheumatoid arthritis, juvenile and pauciarticular are the most common types.

Post-infectious painful joints occur following rheumatic fever, but this is now rare. Allergic phenomena such as Henoch–Schönlein purpura may present with joint pain. Haemorrhagic disorders such as haemophilia can cause long-standing joint disruption, as can leukaemia. Your history taking should be directed at identifying the likely cause, e.g. was there a history of recent viral illness? Is the child known to be haemophiliac? Have there been previous admissions for treatment (suggesting an ongoing, possibly rheumatic origin)?

Your examination should illustrate your concern not to hurt the child, but you should elicit the clinical signs. Remember to check for effusions at the knees.

Other causes of painful joints or limp may be presented. Transient synovitis follows a viral infection, but can be difficult to distinguish from Perthe's disease when the hip is involved.

FACTFILE

1. About 6% of children thought to have transient synovitis develop Perthe's disease.
2. The sequelae of missing the diagnosis of congenital hip dislocation are severe. Babies born by breech delivery are at increased risk.
3. Scoliosis of the spine is a curvature of the spine in the coronal plane; the majority are idiopathic and occur in females.
4. There is no ideal screening test for dislocation of the hip.
5. Accidents are the single greatest contributor to mortality rates in children between the ages of 3 and 14.

DISCUSSION POINTS

1. You must know the available tests for screening for hip dislocation. Ultrasound examination of the hip may become popular, but its role is as yet uncertain although large trials are addressing this.

2. Club foot occurs in around one per 1000 births. Treatment is difficult and prolonged. You should know the different types and the procedures available for management.

3. *Staphylococcus pyogenes* is the commonest organism in osteomyelitis. The diagnostic indicators are important and you should know them. Do not mention X-rays as being initially valuable: only students who have not been around think they are. Radiological changes in acute osteomyelitis are not obvious within the first 10 days of presentation.

4. Know the difference between osteogenesis imperfecta and osteochondritis. For some reason some students confuse these very different conditions.

5. Painful joints may also follow trauma. This can lead on to discussion of topics such as accident prevention in paediatrics. This is an area of increasing importance. Similarly, trauma may not have been that much of an accident and you may end up discussing non-accidental injury and at-risk registers.

AND FINALLY

Repetition of this does no harm: smile at the child and be nice!

QUESTIONS

APGAR SCORES

A1   What are the components of the Apgar score?

A2   Who was Apgar?

ASTHMA

A3   Which household allergens commonly are associated with asthma?

ATOPY

A4   What conditions have an atopic basis?

BILIRUBIN

B1   What are the causes of elevated bilirubin levels in a 1-day-old child?

B2   What are the causes of elevated bilirubin levels in a 12-day-old child?

BREAST MILK

B3   What are the 'active ingredients' of breast milk?

BREATH-HOLDING ATTACKS

B4   At what age do breath-holding attacks occur and how are they treated?

BRONCHIECTASIS

B5   What are the clinical features of bronchiectasis?

BRUISING

B6   What causes of bruising in children do you know of?

CEPHALHAEMATOMA

C1   Where does this haematoma lie anatomically?

CHRISTMAS DISEASE

C2 How is the normal coagulation cascade altered in Christmas disease?

COELIAC DISEASE

C3 How does coeliac disease present?

C4 What investigations should be performed to confirm or refute this diagnosis?

CONVULSIONS

C5 How are febrile convulsions managed and what long-term advice might be given to parents?

DEATH

D1 What are the three commonest causes of death in children between the age of 5 and 14?

DIARRHOEA

D2 How is childhood diarrhoea managed?

DUCHENNE DYSTROPHY

D3 What is the pattern of inheritance of Duchenne muscular dystrophy?

DUODENAL ATRESIA

D4 What chromosomal abnormalities may be associated with duodenal atresia?

ENURESIS

E1 What is the incidence of enuresis in children below 10 years of age?

E2 What effective treatments are available for the management of enuresis in a 5-year-old?

EPILEPSY

E3 What types of epilepsy may be seen in childhood?

ERB'S PALSY

E4   What is Erb's palsy and how is it treated?

FALLOT'S TETRALOGY

F1   What are the cardiac abnormalities in this condition?

FORMULA FEEDS

F2   What is the calorie content of 100 ml of formula feed?

GASTRO-OESOPHAGEAL REFLUX

G1   How might gastro-oesophageal reflux present?

GENETIC DISORDERS

G2   What common genetic disorders do you know?

GLUCOSE-6-PHOSPHATE DEHYDROGENASE

G3   Which drugs should be avoided in people deficient in
         this enzyme?

G4   How might this enzyme deficiency present to
         neonatologists?

GUTHRIE TEST

G5   What is this test used for and what is the principle
         underlying its application?

HAEMATURIA

H1   How should haematuria be assessed in a 6-year-old boy?

HAEMORRHAGIC DISEASE OF THE NEWBORN

H2   What causes this condition and how is it prevented?

HEPATOMEGALY

H3   What are the causes of liver enlargement in children?

HIP

H4   What tests should be used to screen for congenital
         dislocation of the hip?

HIRSCHSPRUNG'S DISEASE

H5 When does Hirschsprung's disease present and how is it managed?

HYDROCEPHALUS

H6 What types of hydrocephalus do you know?

IMMUNIZATION

I1 What immunization schedules should be used in childhood?

INFECTIOUS MONONUCLEOSIS

I2 What is the differential diagnosis of this condition?

INTUSSUSCEPTION

I3 How might this condition be conservatively managed?

JAUNDICE

J1 What infectious conditions cause jaundice?

JOINT PAIN

J2 What are the causes of polyarthropathy in a 6-year-old?

KAWASAKI DISEASE

K1 Which complication of this condition carries a high mortality rate?

KLINEFELTER'S SYNDROME

K2 What long-term problems do boys with this condition experience?

KWASHIORKOR

K3 What is meant by the term kwashiorkor and how common is this condition?

LICE

L1 How are head lice treated?

LYMPHADENOPATHY

L2 What are the commoner causes of generalized lymphadenopathy in childhood?

MESENTERIC ADENITIS

M1 What is the differential diagnosis in a case of mesenteric adenitis?

MICROCEPHALY

M2 What are the causes of microcephaly?

NEPHROBLASTOMA

N1 What is this condition and at what age does it most commonly present?

NEPHROTIC SYNDROME

N2 How might nephrotic syndrome be classified in childhood?

OESOPHAGUS

O1 How does oesophageal atresia present?

ORTOLANI'S TEST

O2 How sensitive is this test?

PERTHE'S DISEASE

P1 What is the sex distribution of Perthe's disease?

PRADER–WILLI SYNDROME

P2 What is this condition?

PREMATURITY

P3 What are the common clinical problems with preterm babies?

QUELLADA

Q1 What is the approved name for this agent and what is it used for?

REHYDRATION

R1 What are the indications for oral rehydration?

REYE'S SYNDROME

R2 What is known about the cause of Reye's syndrome?

SEPTICAEMIA

S1 What clinical signs may be seen in meningococcal septicaemia?

SPLENECTOMY

S2 What are indications for this operation and what advice must be given to parents about child care postoperatively?

THALASSAEMIA

T1 What types of thalassaemia do you know?

TOXOPLASMOSIS

T2 What are the clinical features of congenital toxoplasmosis?

TUBEROUS SCLEROSIS

T3 What pattern of inheritance does this condition demonstrate?

URETHRAL VALVES

U1 Which sex is affected by posterior urethral valves?

VIRAL INFECTIONS

V1 Which viral infections in pregnancy cause neonatal problems?

WARTS

W1 How are plantar warts in children best managed?

X-RAY

X1 What are the radiological features of Perthe's disease?

ZOSTER

Z1 What are the features of the rash in childhood herpes zoster infection?

ANSWERS

A1 Respiratory effort, heart rate, colour, response to stimuli and muscle tone.

A2 Virginia Apgar, obstetric anaesthetist, devised this scoring system in 1953.

A3 House dust mite and moulds.

A4 Many, but asthma, allergic rhinitis and atopic eczema are the most common.

B1 In a 1-day-old infant the principal causes relate to haemolysis, such as rhesus disease, ABO incompatability and to sepsis.

B2 In a 12-day-old child causes such as breastfeeding, hypothyroidism and bile duct obstruction are more likely.

B3 Cells, enzymes (lipase) lysozymes and immunoglobulins etc.

B4 Usually 1–3 years. Parental reassurance.

B5 Cough and finger clubbing.

B6 Accidents and non-accidental injury. Haemophilia, Christmas disease, Von Willebrand's disease, idiopathic thrombocytopenic purpura and Henoch–Schönlein purpura.

C1 Subperiosteal.

C2 Factor IX deficiency.

C3 Failure to thrive. Occasionally with hypocalcaemia.

C4 Diagnosis is by jejunal biopsy following challenge with gluten. Testing for antigliadin and anti-endomysial antibodies, though not diagnostic, is useful for screening.

C5 Parents should be advised to keep the child cool and treat with paracetamol. The risk of developing epilepsy is small but the risk of recurrence of another febrile convulsion is around 30%.

D1 Accident, malignancy and infection.

D2 Oral rehydration is the primary treatment. In very young children breast or formula feeding should be reintroduced early.

D3 X-linked recessive.

D4 Trisomy 21 accounts for one-third of these cases.

E1 Incidence is around 15% at 5 years of age and 3% among 10-year-olds.

E2 Reassurance of both parents and child is helpful and a variety of approaches have been used, including alarm systems activated by a sensor pad becoming wet and nasal/oral desmopressin.

E3 The types of epilepsy in childhood are generally the same as those seen in the adult population, and should be classified into generalized and partial seizures.

E4 Brachial plexus damage at C5–6. The treatment consists of gentle physiotherapy.

F1 Ventricular septal defect, pulmonary stenosis, overriding aorta and right ventricular hypertrophy.

F2 67 kCal.

G1 Irritability, vomiting, haematemesis, 'apnoeic episodes' and failure to thrive.

G2 Trisomies such as 21, 18 and 13. Single gene disorders such as cystic fibrosis and the inborn errors of metabolism. Polygenic disorders such as neural tube defect.

G3 Aspirin, sulphonamides.

G4 May present as neonatal jaundice in male infants of Asian origin.

G5 Diagnosis of phenylketonuria. It is a test based upon bacterial inhibition.

H1 Thoroughly! Urinalysis, urine culture and microscopy and renal imaging, including ultrasound. Blood should be taken for measurement of plasma urea and electrolytes, calcium, phosphate, albumin, full blood count, coagulation screen and sickle cell screen.

H2 Vitamin K deficiency. It is prevented by oral or intramuscular vitamin K.

H3 Remember that the liver is palpable two finger-breadths below the costal margin in infants and young children. The causes include infection, such as hepatitis, infectious mononucleosis and malaria. Cardiovascular causes include any cause of cardiac failure. Other less common causes include lymphomas, leukaemia, storage disorders and haemoglobinopathies.

H4 Ortolani and Barlow's manoeuvres.

H5 Usually in the neonatal period, but may appear later. Management is surgical, involving a colostomy followed by resection of the aganglionic segment. Later anastomosis of normal bowel to the anus may be possible.

H6 Communicating and non-communicating.

I1 It is important to appreciate that immunization schedules occasionally change. You should be aware of the most recent recommendations. An important point is that there are very few contraindications to immunization in childhood. The 'Green Book', properly called *Immunization Against Infectious Disease,* is published regularly by HMSO and covers issues relating to immunization in a comprehensive fashion. The most recent edition was published in 1996.

I2   The clinical features of glandular fever in young children are non-specific. The lymphadenopathy in older children may suggest a diagnosis of lymphoma or leukaemia.

I3   Usually by air enema, though reduction by barium enema is still used.

J1   Hepatitis viruses, CMV, EBV etc.

J2   Juvenile rheumatoid arthritis and postviral infection.

K1   Coronary artery aneurysms.

K2   Infertility, hypogonadism and gynaecomastia in adolescence.

K3   Protein/calorie malnutrition of infants weaned late and fed a high-starch diet. Incidence varies from country to country and on background conditions of population nutrition and civil war!

L1   0.5% malathion is applied to the scalp and dead nits are removed 12 hours later.

L2   Most commonly this is associated with viral infection, but multiple small nodes are commonly found in the neck, axillae and inguinal area of small children. Much less commonly, lymphadenopathy may be caused by leukaemia or lymphoma.

M1   The chief differential diagnosis is appendicitis. It is important also to remember that abdominal pain in children may be the presenting feature of pneumonia, and occasionally of diabetes.

M2 Microcephaly may be subsequent to perinatal hypoxia or infection such as meningitis, resulting in reduced brain substance. Congenital infection and genetic disorders are also associated with microcephaly. In a proportion of cases the condition is familial.

N1 Also called Wilm's tumour, this is a malignancy originating in embryonic renal tissue and usually presents in children of 5 or younger.

N2 Nephrotic syndrome is classified as steroid-sensitive nephrotic syndrome, steroid-resistant nephrotic syndrome and congenital nephrotic syndrome.

O1 This may present during pregnancy as polyhydramnios or, postnatally, as persistent salivation associated with choking and cyanotic episodes, particularly after feeds.

O2 Around six cases per 1000 births are identified by clinical testing. Further examination confirms the disease in only 1.5 cases per 1000 births.

P1 Male to female ratio is 5:1.

P2 A genetic disorder characterized by developmental delay, obesity and hypogonadism.

P3 Respiratory distress syndrome, persistent fetal circulation, apnoea, necrotizing enterocolitis, retinopathy of prematurity and problems of nutrition.

Q1 Lindane. Scabies.

R1 Mild dehydration, i.e. no clinical evidence of dehydration but vomiting and diarrhoea continuing and weight loss less than 5% of body weight. More serious dehydration requires intravenous therapy.

R2   The cause of this encephalopathy is unknown, but there is a clear association with aspirin and its incidence has fallen following the reduction in the use of aspirin in children below 12 years.

S1   Collapse associated with a purpuric rash, which is irregular in outline and may have a necrotic centre. Septicaemia may occur without meningitis, and carries a worse prognosis.

S2   Steroid-resistant immune thrombocytopenic purpura and trauma are the main indications. Pneumococcal vaccination is advocated.

T1   Alpha-thalassaemia and beta-thalassaemia. The latter is further classified as major and minor.

T2   The chief features are retinopathy, hydrocephaly, hepatomegaly and anaemia.

T3   Autosomal dominant, but most cases are new mutations.

U1   Males. Look for a poor urine stream and a palpable bladder.

V1   Rubella and cytomegalovirus are the principal viral teratogens.

W1   Most disappear and do not actually require treatment.

X1   Flattening and fragmentation of the femoral head epiphysis.

Z1   The same as in adults, although pain is not such a feature.